Praise for

FOOD BABE
family

This is not your average cookbook. This is like having Vani by your side in the kitchen to help you feed your family delicious, healthy, real food. Vani has a passion for telling the truth about what we eat and busting food myths—all while offering practical and delicious alternatives. From healthy school lunches to weeknight dinners everyone can get excited about, she'll help you feed your family simple, healthy, real food.

— **Gabby Bernstein**, #1 *New York Times* best-selling
author of *The Universe Has Your Back*

Finally, a comprehensive guide to the grocery store, fridge, pantry, and kitchen serving up the knowledge that can keep our children safe from the hidden harms in our food system. All the while providing fun and delicious recipes that will delight their picky palates. Vani Hari has done it again with *Food Babe Family*. Every parent and grandparent needs to read and follow her advice to raise healthy, focused children.

— **Mark Hyman, MD**, author of the #1 *New York Times* bestseller *Young Forever*

Vani is my go-to expert for transparency in the food industry. *Food Babe Family* has all the hot tips and advice to inspire any kid to love real food from day one. Vani is a wealth of knowledge when it comes to family food and the recipes throughout are drool-worthy. Every parent needs this book in their arsenal.

— **Catherine McCord**, entrepreneur, author, and founder of Weelicious + One Potato

Food Babe Family is a powerful resource for all parents. Vani removes many of the obstacles we parents experience trying to navigate the best ways to institute healthy eating for our children. I appreciate that she doesn't make it about "healthy eating" but a natural way to make this a lifestyle for you and your children. There are enough recipes to cater to every family's preferences, and as a bonus, she arms you with the tools to navigate the grocery store. I admire Vani's continued commitment to helping us all live and eat better.

— **Gabby Reece**, *New York Times* best-selling author and host
of the #1 mental health podcast *The Gabby Reece Show*

FOOD BABE *family*

ALSO BY VANI HARI

*Feeding You Lies**

The Food Babe Way

*Food Babe Kitchen**

*Available from Hay House

Please visit:

Hay House USA: www.hayhouse.com®
Hay House Australia: www.hayhouse.com.au
Hay House UK: www.hayhouse.co.uk
Hay House India: www.hayhouse.co.in

FOOD BABE

BABE

family

More Than 100 Recipes and Foolproof Strategies to Help Your Kids Fall in Love with Real Food

VANI HARI

HAY HOUSE LLC

Carlsbad, California • New York City
London • Sydney • New Delhi

Published in the United States by: Hay House LLC: www.hayhouse.com®
Published in Australia by: Hay House Australia Publishing Pty Ltd: www.hayhouse.com.au
Published in the United Kingdom by: Hay House UK Ltd: www.hayhouse.co.uk
Published in India by: Hay House Publishers (India) Pvt Ltd: www.hayhouse.co.in

Indexer: Joan Shapiro
Cover and Interior design: Julie Davison
Lifestyle photography: Susan Stripling
Recipe stylist and photography: Kim Ruggles

Library of Congress Control Number: 2023940126

Tradepaper ISBN: 978-1-4019-7600-2
E-book ISBN: 978-1-4019-7408-4

10 9 8 7 6 5 4 3 2 1
1st edition, October 2023
2nd edition, April 2025

Printed in China

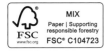

To my children, Harley
and Finley (Bru).
May your love of real food
inspire everyone around you.
You are the greatest gift
I have ever received;
thank you for all your love.

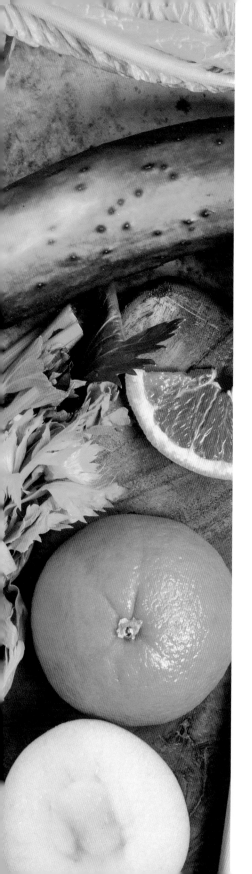

CONTENTS

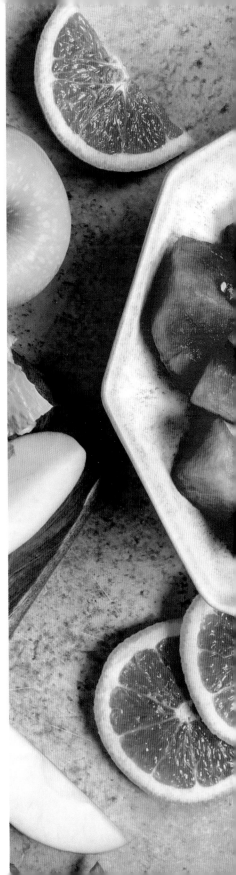

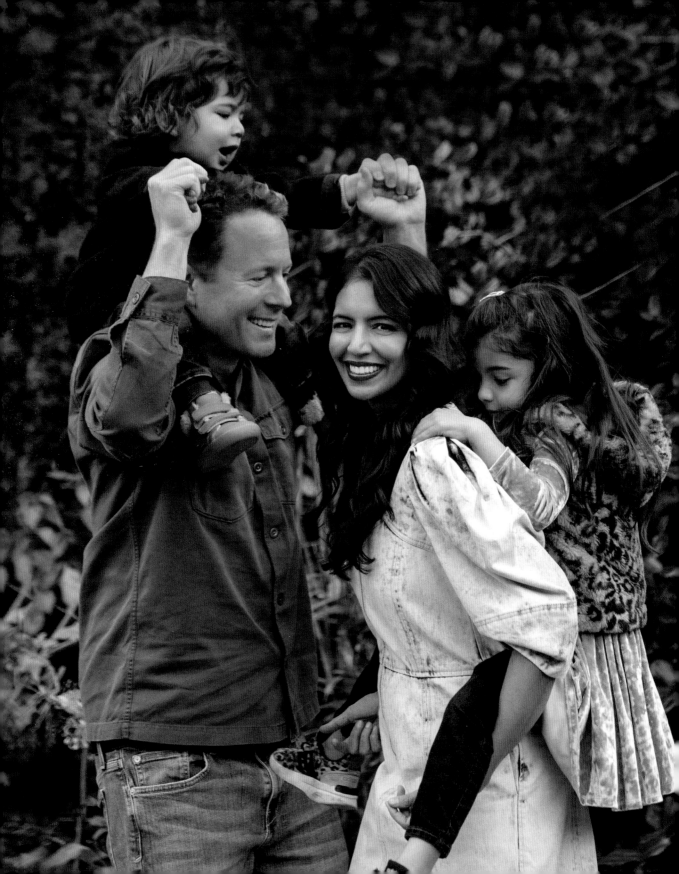

INTRODUCTION

I was at my daughter's school, waiting for the parent orientation meeting to start, and I hadn't felt this nervous in a long time. In a few weeks, my daughter Harley would be eating lunch at school for the first time, and I was trying to figure out how I was going to address a burning issue that had been on my mind for months: Pizza Fridays.

Over the past year, when I picked up Harley from preschool, I had noticed that every Friday there was a pizza delivery from Domino's. As a food activist, author, and investigator of what's in our food, I knew the ingredients in Domino's pizzas were not ones that I would wish to go into my little girl's body every Friday. At the same time, I didn't want my daughter to miss out on the social aspect of Pizza Fridays. This school meeting was the perfect time to discuss this conflicted feeling; but honestly, I was worried about how everyone was going to react. Would the teachers think I was being difficult? Would the other parents be upset and think I was going to ruin their easy day off from making lunch?

As the Q&A session started, I became even more anxious but didn't want to miss my opportunity. One parent beat me to the punch: "Please bring back Pizza Fridays!" they cried out. I knew this was the opening I needed, so I followed up with, "Will there be an opportunity to possibly change where we get our pizza from? Because there are several questionable ingredients in Domino's, one being TBHQ that affects children's immune systems."

I knew TBHQ would be the best ingredient to mention. Parents will do anything to keep kids from getting sick (and giving that sickness to everyone in the house). So I was hoping this would get the attention of the parents in the room. Indeed, I immediately felt tension in the air.

After a moment, the headmaster responded with uncertainty, saying they had tried another pizza place in the past and the kids did not like it as much. I noticed some other parents nod in agreement.

So when school started, I sent the headmaster my research on Domino's and made a case for change. I felt a little defeated by her response, which was about costs. Domino's was pretty cheap! They were charging about seven bucks a pie. How in the world was I going to find a clean pizza place that would match those prices?

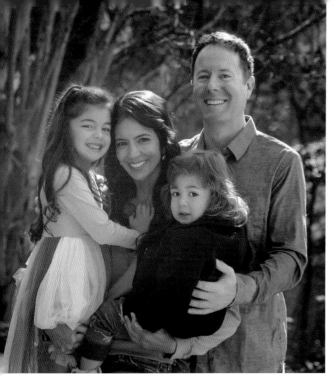

Even though I knew it would be a challenge to meet the monetary constraints I was given, I decided to call several pizza places that used better ingredients. First I called my favorite spot in town, Pure Pizza, which used organic ingredients. I explained my situation and that Domino's was being served at my daughter's school to the owner, Juli Ghazi, and her reaction was, "*Yuck*." I told her my heart would absolutely explode with happiness if my daughter and her classmates were able to eat her pizza instead. I was floored at her response. She was overjoyed to kick Domino's to the curb and match the price, plus free delivery.

The headmaster at Harley's school agreed to make the transition from Domino's to Pure Pizza. I was on cloud nine after I heard the news!

Throughout this whole process, I had been sharing my findings with Harley—giving her little updates here and there, whether at the dinner table or during our nightly chats before bed. She was stoked!

I shared what happened with Harley's pediatrician, Dr. Ana Maria Temple, at Harley's annual checkup. She gave me a high five. She asked me if she could contact the owner of Pure Pizza and the school's headmaster because she wanted to let them know how heroic this decision was. In her note to the headmaster, she said:

I am writing to thank you for your willingness to work with Pure Pizza and bring children real ingredients and real food for Pizza Friday . . . I am a holistic pediatrician in town, and for the past 14 years I have been educating kids and families in various schools and on social media about how food impacts learning. Times are changing, but there is still a lot of resistance out there surrounding food ingredients and health consequences. At times I feel like I am trying to convert people to a new religion. Thank you for being a pioneer in changing Pizza Friday to a wholesome affair. I hope more schools follow your example.

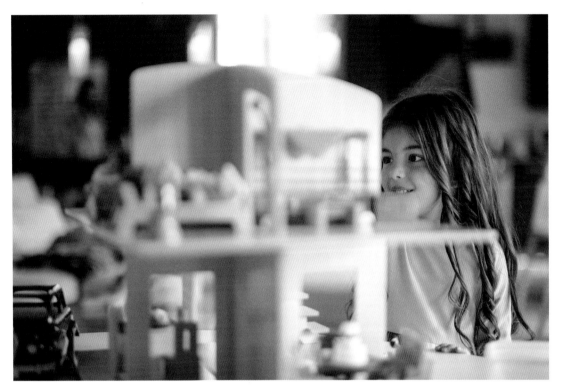

This is why I do what I do.

Hi, I'm Vani Hari, also known as the Food Babe. I'm a food activist who's gotten giant food companies like Kraft and Subway to change their food, a *New York Times* best-selling author of three books, and the co-owner of Truvani, an organic product brand. I used to be sick, on several prescription drugs, and overweight; I felt like a zombie for most of my life, until I found real food. I have a passion for telling everyone the truth about what's in our food. I want everyone to feel as good as I do now!

Since becoming a mom, my dedication to healthy eating has skyrocketed. Passing down everything I have learned about food to my children has been such a joy, and teaching them why what we eat matters is my number-one priority. As they grow, I'm teaching my kids the truth about where our food comes from and how to make food choices as carefully as I do (age appropriately, of course). Over the last few years, I've thrown myself into researching how our lives have been hijacked by Big Food companies who lure children in, coaxing them with targeted marketing into craving processed and sugary foods from a very early age. This process begins within the first year of life, and it accelerates as soon as they are able to start asking for processed snacks like Disney princess Goldfish crackers and Scooby Doo Fruit Snacks. Sadly, this has created multiple generations of children who are hooked on ultra-processed packaged foods, and who end up being "picky eaters" later in life. Big

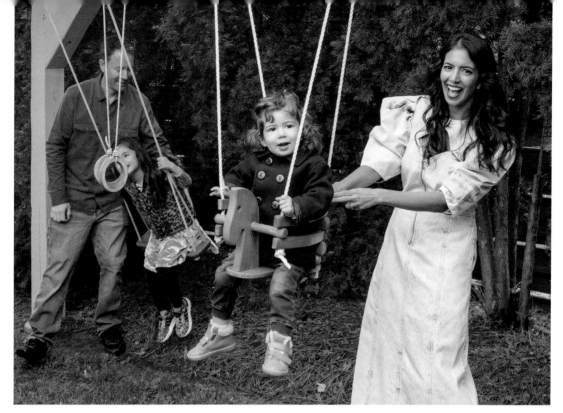

Food's influence is one of several reasons why many children don't like to eat vegetables; likewise, I believe this is a major reason why obesity, type 2 diabetes, and cancer rates are steadily rising in children across America.[1] Thankfully, it doesn't need to be this way.

I've learned how to shun the overly processed fast-food world—not just for myself, but for my children too. The Big Food industry has used their vast resources to target parents, convincing them that it's difficult to feed their children good food. But here's the truth: Parenting is difficult, but feeding your children simple, healthy, real food shouldn't be. In this book, I provide you with all the tools, information, and recipes you need to feed your children in a way that will foster a love for real food and set them up for a life of healthy eating. Let me preface this by saying that I'm not a childhood feeding expert. I'm also not a nutritionist or registered dietician. Everything I've learned and shared in this book is based on my own independent research and consulting with experts after I became sick (pun intended) of processed food and set out to create a change in my life.

This book you are holding is much more than your average family cookbook. I couldn't simply leave you with recipes without showing you all the ins and outs of our life as a Food Babe Family. In the first section of this book, I'll recount a typical day in our household as I prepare food for my children. I will dispel some great myths we have been fed about feeding children and help you spot ridiculous product marketing. You will learn how to navigate many sticky food situations that you will undoubtedly encounter at birthday parties, restaurants, and while traveling. I'll give you the play-by-play on how to pack yummy school lunches that your children will love. I'll give you healthy store-bought swaps for ultra-processed snacks so that your children don't feel like they're missing out.

The second half of this book provides over 100 delicious and simple recipes to make the process of feeding your family even easier! Because I believe that no one should have anxiety when feeding their children.

Don't feel like you need to start at the beginning and read this book through like it's a novel. Start with the sections that interest you the most, and those that apply to what you are currently struggling with. Think of this as the ultimate reference book for helping your child develop a love for real food in any situation or stage in their life.

You may find some of my advice unconventional. The "real food" lifestyle is certainly different from how most parents have been told to feed their children; but for my family, it works. The purpose of this book is to share how I personally feed my family and the challenges we face when surrounded by processed food temptations. I want to assure you that we don't feel deprived. Quite the opposite! Living without processed food is so rewarding. We enjoy our mealtimes together, eat a wide variety of incredibly delicious food, and have a great routine that keeps us on track. Our children are learning remarkably healthy eating habits (they love vegetables and fresh food from the earth), and I hope they will keep this love for real food throughout their lives.

Above all else, please don't feel overwhelmed. The habits and routines we follow work for my family, but they may not be for everyone. If you take just one tidbit of advice from this book that helps you and your family eat healthier, this could very well snowball and grow into much bigger changes in the future. Start with what works for you and see what happens next.

Together, we can help undo the damage done by the multibillion-dollar processed food industry over the last 100 years. Maybe someday, we can even put a stop to their unethical marketing campaigns that target our kids with products full of harmful ingredients. Our children are the future. Setting them up with the tools they need to thrive in a world that is overloaded with fast, easy junk food full of health-wrecking ingredients is a practice that's worth its weight in gold.

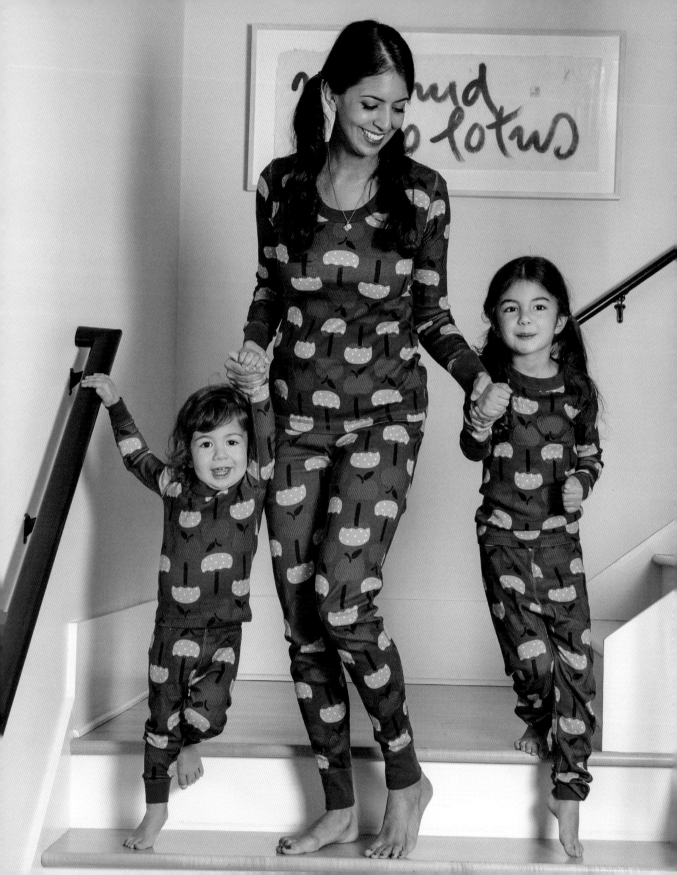

PART I

LIVE LIKE A FOOD BABE FAMILY

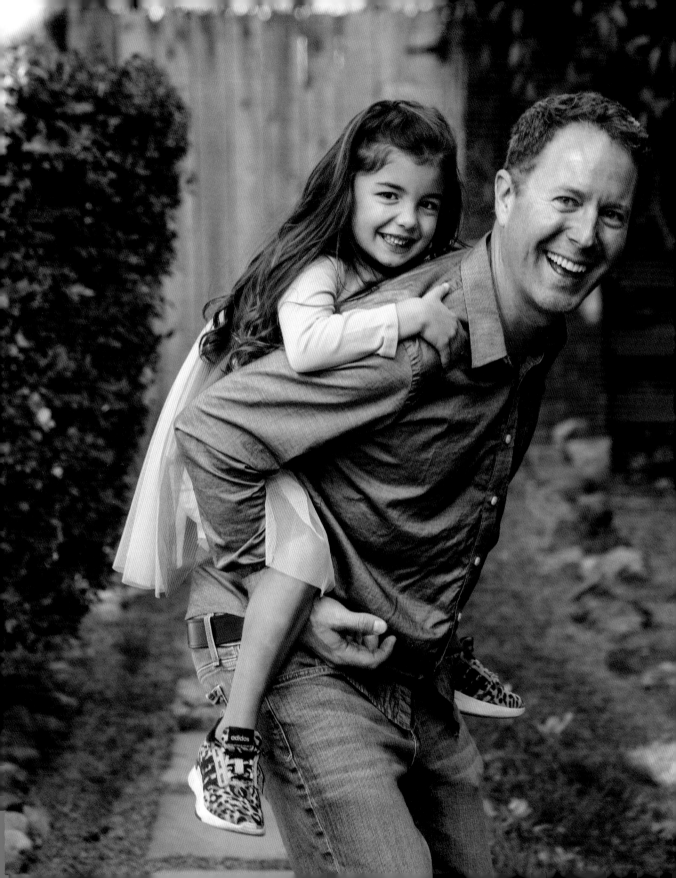

chapter 1

RAISING CHILDREN TO LOVE REAL FOOD

WHY SOME CHILDREN HATE VEGETABLES

When my daughter started eating solid food, I didn't buy any jarred or packaged "baby food." That's right: I never bought a single jar of pureed peas, pureed bananas—pureed anything. I didn't buy squeeze packs and puffs. I didn't buy rice cereal. I also didn't blend fruits and veggies at home to make my own homemade "baby food." Right about now you may be wondering what in the world I *did* feed my daughter.

The truth is that feeding babies and children is not complicated, and you don't need the vast majority of these packaged baby foods, puffs, bars, and squeeze pouches. These are your child's earliest forms of processed food, and sadly, eating a processed

food diet is the number-one reason why many kids don't like vegetables later in life.

This is not meant to be a slap in the face. I need to share the truth with you about foods that are marketed toward babies and toddlers, but I'm not here to shame you. If you've been buying and feeding your child the foods I warn about in this chapter, please don't feel like you've done anything wrong. Parenting isn't easy, and I know you want the best for your child. There is a multibillion-dollar industry out there that uses their vast resources to target advertising to you, coaxing you into believing that you need these products to be "good" parents.

Children can start with regular whole foods, as long as they are prepared (sometimes straight from your own plate) into soft finger foods. This approach is called

Baby-Led Weaning, a concept that was first introduced to me in a book by Gill Rapley and Tracey Murkett, *Baby-Led Weaning: The Essential Guide to Introducing Solid Foods and Helping Your Baby to Grow Up a Happy and Confident Eater.*

The first solid food I fed to both of my children was avocado. I started with avocado because it typically doesn't cause allergic reactions, has a mild flavor, and is full of nutrients, good fats, and calories. It's also soft and easy for babies to eat. It makes the perfect first food! Of course, avocado is technically a fruit, but it is not sweet. It's important to create a savory palate in your child instead of fostering a preference that everything be sweet—most of your baby's food shouldn't be sweet or sugary. It's much easier to promote a love for savory food from the start than it is to break a sugar addiction later in life.

Introducing Vegetables as Baby's First Solid Food

When my youngest, Finley, reached about six months old, I could see that he was ready to start eating solid food. He wanted to be at the table when we all sat down to eat and get a plate of his own. All babies are different, and when they are ready to start on solid food varies; you'll know that it's time when they become very interested in what you are eating and watch you intently while you eat or start grabbing at your fork. They'll also be able to sit on their own and hold their head up with good control. It's been shown that there is a short window of time when babies are most receptive to new foods—somewhere between four to seven months old. (But this time frame can increase when babies are exposed to a wide variety of tastes and textures as early as possible.)

When Finley seemed ready for his first solid food, I mashed avocado with some water. He really liked it. I fed this to him once per day for three days in a row before moving on to any other foods. I paired this with breastfeeding on demand, which was about seven times a day at the time. I introduced one food at a time for three days so that I could monitor for any negative reactions or allergies. After those first three days of just avocado and breast milk, I added a little extra virgin olive oil to his avocado mash. I monitored him again for any reactions, and he responded beautifully.

Then it was time to introduce another food. I moved on to carrots. I steamed the carrots in sticks that were big enough for him to hold, but not so round or big that they'd pose a choking hazard. He loved these too. After three days of plain carrots, I added a little grass-fed butter to them, and he ate them all up!

I continued going down a list of vegetables to feed Finley every three days. Next up was zucchini, which he loves with grass-fed butter. This was one of his early favorites. I can't say the same for green beans, which he at first just played with and then threw on the floor; but after reintroducing them a few times, they're now one of his favorite vegetables. Which brings me to a very important point: Children don't always like new foods the first time they taste them. Perhaps not even the second or the third time. In fact, it's been shown that children sometimes need

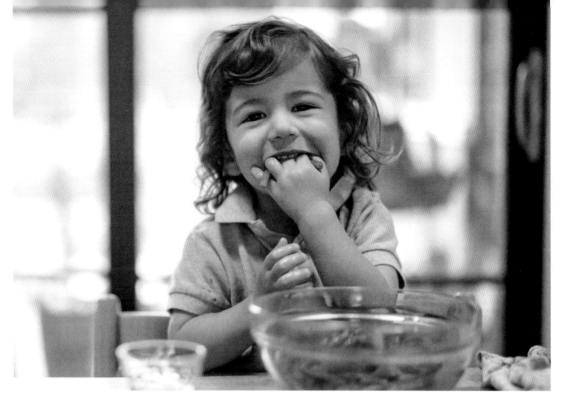

to be offered a new food as many as 10 to 15 times before they will eat it.[1] So, don't give up. And don't worry: it's common for babies to make funny facial expressions when they first experience new flavors, such as fruity, sour, and bitter. Think about a time when you've seen a baby suck on a slice of lemon and they distort their face in disgust. That disgusted face doesn't mean they don't like lemons! It just means that they are experiencing sour for one of the first times in their life—it's a natural reaction. The same goes for bitter foods like broccoli and even those dreaded green beans that Finley kept throwing on the floor. Many parents give up after one or two rejections of a new food, but I'm here to tell you not to throw in the towel so quickly. Keep offering good foods to your baby and you will both discover what they love in time. Every child takes to solid food

differently and will go at their own pace. When I started to feed Harley solid foods, she didn't eat very much. Now she is a great eater. It's an entirely different story with Finley! He was bigger and ate a whole lot more as a baby. So, just start slowly and your child will let you know when they are ready to move on.

How Soon Is Too Soon for Veggies?

Experts say it's best to start introducing vegetables right when babies begin eating solids—and continue offering them vegetables at every meal, no matter what. Remember, babies are most receptive to new tastes between four and seven months of age,[2] so you don't want to miss the boat! You can do this without having to resort to jarred and packaged food. When very young children eat packaged foods they are reinforcing a love for sweet and heavily processed foods instead of for the healthiest foods on our planet: vegetables.

One thing I'm not a fan of is mixing different fruits, vegetables, or grains into one puree. For example, if I wanted to serve sweet potatoes, I mashed sweet potatoes with grass-fed butter. I kept each food separated, so that Finley learned what each specific food tasted like—and learned to love real food that is prepared simply. If I had mixed it with apple (as you find in some store-bought purees or squeeze packs), the taste would differ from that of a simple sweet potato. Finley learned quickly that he loves zucchini, but perhaps not beets. We wouldn't have figured this out if I'd blended them together.

The majority of packaged baby food is mixed with fruit, to make it sweet and more palatable for young children who aren't accustomed to bitter tastes. For example, Gerber sells jars of "Apple Zucchini Peach" and "Apple Spinach Kale" purees. Admittedly, I have never tasted these products, but I'll venture a guess that they taste mostly like sweet apples and nothing like bitter zucchini, kale, or spinach. Beech-Nut and many organic brands make similar purees and pouches filled with zucchini and kale blended with sweet fruits. The children eating these products are getting some vegetables into their diet, but they are not experiencing the actual bitter taste of them. How is your child expected to love zucchini if they have never tasted it? Sadly, if they don't experience it at a young age, it may be an uphill battle for them to like zucchini (or other bitter vegetables) as they grow older. This is why I believe it's best to give babies plain vegetables from the get-go. Perhaps add some grass-fed butter when they're ready for it.

This isn't just common sense; it's backed by science. According to researchers at the University of Colorado School of Medicine, a big reason kids don't seem to like green vegetables is because they are not nurtured to like the flavor and bitterness of them from a young age.[3] While babies naturally love sweets, they need to be exposed to dark green vegetables on a regular basis to learn to love them. The researchers further found that a major contributor to the problem was all these prepared baby foods out there that don't prominently contain vegetables. Out of 548 foods reviewed, they found that only 52 of them were single-vegetable products and *none* of those were simply dark green vegetables.

Let Mealtime Be a Messy Time!

At this stage, you want your baby to get really comfortable with the food you are giving them, so let them be messy and play with their food. Allow them to smear it around and smoosh some in their hair. It's natural for babies to taste something and then spit it out. Remember, this doesn't mean they'll never love it; they are just getting to know a new taste. This is a learning time for babies to feel, taste, and smell this new food, and to get used to it. It's been shown that babies who are allowed to play with their food are less picky and have fewer food aversions later in life.

At first I did what most parents do, and gave Finley a sippy cup as his first cup for his water. I always give him water with solid food, but quickly realized that I hated that plastic sippy cup after day two and threw it in my donation pile. I avoid plastic as much as possible because it can contain endocrine disruptors and other chemicals that can be harmful to health. I also wanted to train his lips to drink from a real cup versus an artificial plastic spout. I decided to teach him to drink water from a tempered glass cup without a lid, and started doing so when he was only six months old. I helped him, and yes, there were accidents, but it was only water so it cleaned up easily.

Moving beyond Fruits and Vegetables

Finley's first food that wasn't a fruit or vegetable was an organic pastured egg yolk. I would boil the egg and mash the yolk with olive oil or grass-fed butter. Egg yolks are great for babies if they can tolerate them. To start, you should only feed them the yolk, because this part of the egg doesn't contain the proteins that are associated with allergic reactions.[4] Also, it's been shown that when you introduce eggs to babies between four and six months old (versus when they are over a year old) they are less likely to develop egg allergies later in life.[5] Pastured egg yolk is a good source of DHA and B vitamins, and it is high in choline, which supports nutrient absorption, good liver function, and memory development. Egg yolks

are also a natural source of absorbable iron, which babies need for brain development.

For decades, parents have been told that rice cereal is the perfect first food, but I believe this is a bunch of B.S. Why is that? Read on.

FIRST FOOD RED FLAG: BEWARE OF RICE CEREALS

The following probably goes against everything you've heard about how great rice cereal is for babies, but this is Big Food's marketing engine at work. One reason rice cereal is recommended for babies is because it is supposedly a great source of iron for babies. The package of Gerber Rice Cereal says that it contains iron to "help support learning ability." So, it must be good for them, right?

The truth is that processed white rice flour, the primary ingredient in rice cereal, doesn't contain iron. It has no nutrition in it naturally, so it's artificially "fortified" with synthetic iron called ferrous fumarate. This doesn't make rice cereal a good source of iron. There's ample evidence that our bodies do not absorb and process synthetic nutrients as well as the nutrients found in real whole foods. It's much healthier to get your nutrients from whole foods, including your iron from real foods like grass-fed meats, eggs, and leafy greens. And this goes for babies and children too.

But wait. There is a much more important reason why you should be wary of rice cereals.

Arsenic Abounds in Rice Products

Arsenic is one dangerous substance that you don't want to be feeding to your baby, especially during this crucial time in their life while their brains are still developing. Even small amounts of arsenic can threaten the neurological development of babies and toddlers, and the effects may be irreversible. Arsenic accumulates in the body, so the risk increases the more often your child is exposed. Arsenic is a heavy metal that is naturally occurring in the environment, so it sometimes ends up in our food, and because of the way rice is grown, it's often a big culprit for arsenic contamination. This can be very scary as a parent when you realize that many of your baby's earliest foods are rice based, such as rice cereal, teething biscuits, and puffs.

In 2018, Consumer Reports[6] tested baby and toddler foods from the grocery store, and found alarming amounts of heavy metals in the majority of the products. Shockingly, every single product had measurable levels, and nearly two-thirds of the products were contaminated with "worrisome levels" of at least one: arsenic, lead, or cadmium. The most contaminated foods were found to be those containing rice and other rice-based ingredients (like brown rice syrup)—they all contained excessive levels of arsenic and other heavy metals. Sadly, organic products were found to have the same contaminants, so choosing organic does not always protect you.

After this testing was done, Consumer Reports asked Walmart, Gerber, Plum Organics, Happy Family Organics, and Hain Celestial to suspend sales of their infant rice cereals because of consistently high arsenic levels found in these products.[7] Walmart indicated that they would stop selling Parent's Choice rice cereal in their stores, but would continue to sell Gerber and Earth's Best rice cereals. Earth's Best and Gerber continued selling their rice cereals, claiming that they had taken steps to reduce the amount of arsenic in these products.

Although brands have been put on notice about the high levels of arsenic often found in rice, this problem continues. In 2021, Beech-Nut issued a recall of its Single Grain Rice Cereal after routine testing in Alaska found arsenic levels that exceeded recent FDA guidance.[8] This just goes to show that companies need to be doing more to test their products on a regular basis to ensure that they aren't laden with harmful arsenic.

Consumer Reports tested rice cereals again in 2022 to see if arsenic levels had truly dropped in the most popular brands on the market.[9] What they found was disappointing:

- Gerber Single Grain Infant Rice Cereal averaged 62.9 ppb inorganic arsenic.

- Earth's Best Organic Infant Rice Cereal averaged 66.4 ppb inorganic arsenic.

- Gerber Organic Single Grain Infant Rice Cereal averaged 61.1 ppb inorganic arsenic.

These amounts were lower than in previous tests and within the FDA limit of 100 ppb for total inorganic arsenic in infant rice cereals. However, the average amount of arsenic is still high and greater than what many experts recommend for babies. Arsenic builds up in the body and is linked to behavioral problems, ADHD, lower IQ, and other health issues. It's a safer choice to go with other whole grains when feeding your baby, such as quinoa or oatmeal. However, keep in mind that while oatmeal and quinoa are healthy foods, they don't make great first foods for babies. They simply aren't as nutrient dense as vegetables and fruits. Organic whole grains are better when your child is a little older and you can serve them as part of a complete meal.

JARRED BABY FOOD IS ACTUALLY A PROCESSED FOOD

Before you buy your next jar of pureed peas, consider the idea these are not the same as mashed up peas on a plate. Dr. Jonathan Aviv, author of *The Acid Watcher Diet*,[10] has studied the ingredients and composition of jarred baby food and discovered that even organic versions are surprisingly acidic compared to whole foods. For instance, a jar of banana baby food contains the additives citric acid or ascorbic acid, and according to Dr. Aviv this can transform the entire jar of food so that it is 100 times more acidic than a regular banana. This increased acidity can have an effect on digestion and may give your baby acid reflux. Isn't it just as easy to mash a fresh banana or pear? Please

check your apple sauce ingredients: ascorbic acid is found in some of the best brands, even organic ones. Choose one-ingredient apple sauce; the label should say "organic apple puree."

Look Out for Heavy Metals!

In 2021, a congressional report found that some popular baby foods made by brands like Earth's Best, Gerber, Beech-Nut, and HappyBaby, contained toxic heavy metals (arsenic, lead, cadmium, and mercury) at levels that have the potential to harm babies' neurological development and long-term brain function.[11] Sadly, this goes for organic brands too. The FDA recently proposed guidelines to limit the amount of lead in processed foods intended for babies and young children under two years old, which have not been finalized at the time of this writing. The FDA doesn't currently have regulations that limit heavy metals in most baby foods, so companies are free to continue selling these products with no labels or warnings to the public.

Remember that arsenic isn't added to food; it's a naturally occurring contaminant. This is why you need to know which foods often contain arsenic in large amounts, so you can limit them and be careful where you source them from. Baby and toddler products with the highest levels of arsenic are generally those that contain rice or juice. So, it's a good idea to avoid baby foods with any rice-based ingredients (brown rice, white rice, brown rice syrup, etc.) or juices such as apple juice concentrate.

Are Squeeze Pouches Healthy?

A lot of parents love squeeze pouches where babies can suck food directly from a package, and I can see why. They are super convenient to travel with, don't require a spoon, and kids love them. They also have simple ingredient lists, and organic varieties are easy to find.

From a very young age, children develop habits and start to form opinions about food. Ask yourself this question: *Is squeezing pureed pear into your mouth from a sanitary pouch with a spout the same as picking up pieces of fresh pear and putting them in your mouth?*

Of course it's totally different! When you eat a real pear, you can see it. You can feel the juicy texture in your fingers and smell it. This helps you to learn more about what you are eating and learn to love real food (versus food that comes in a shiny package with a cartoon character on it). When babies see pears in the grocery store, they will start to associate them with the real pears they have been eating at home. If they've been sucking pears through a pouch, it's unlikely they'll make that connection. Offering real whole foods (whenever possible) is how you help foster a love for real food, for life.

More reasons to stop buying squeeze pouches:

- These products typically contain less fiber and more sugar than whole foods, meaning they have an increased ability to spike blood sugar.

- Some pouches have added sugar in the form of "fruit juice concentrate," making the fruit in the pouch sweeter than the real thing.

- They can be highly acidic, just like jarred baby foods, when they have citric acid and ascorbic acid added to them.

- Many are preserved with lemon juice or citric acid, both of which can be harmful to your baby's teeth when they are sucked from a pouch and allowed to sit on the teeth for an extended period.

- Babies and toddlers are developing their fine motor skills, including how to hold food, bring it to their mouths, and chew it. These pouches totally bypass this process, especially the act of chewing.

- Even if the ingredients are simple, these pouches are not as nutrient dense as whole real food and not something to rely on regularly.

I know this is a lot of information to take in. But remember: it's not all or nothing. Parenting is hard work, and no one should have anxiety about feeding their children. I'm all for allowing babies to eat independently, *but* I'm also not against feeding children homemade purees with a loaded teaspoon. I don't typically buy my children squeeze pouches, but I picked up some organic ones by Once Upon a Farm and Serenity Kids for a recent trip—and they were very handy while traveling. It's not all or nothing.

Most of all, remember that the food industry has made it complicated to feed your baby, and it shouldn't be. Feed them simple whole foods. Vegetables at first, moving on to fruits and whole grains like oatmeal, and some meat and dairy if that is part of your own diet. As they get a bit older, they can eat what you eat. Whether you are at home or in a restaurant, you can simply smush up some of the healthy food from your plate and offer it to your child. You are eating good food, so they are eating good food. Don't make this more complicated than it needs to be!

TODDLER FOODS

Teaching my children to love real food has been one of my highlights as a mom. From the very start, I've had so much fun introducing as many vegetables as possible to my children and teaching them about where their food comes from. Thankfully, my husband loves to garden, so we have a huge organic garden at home—we grow everything from goji berries to bok choy. The kids love picking fresh produce, and I know that activity has reinforced their love of real food. We also visit farms in the spring and fall to pick fresh produce and see farm animals.

This is very different from how many young children are exposed to food in their earliest years. The majority of children and babies are being fed out of jars, boxes, and squeeze pouches. The Big Food industry has taken the lead in telling parents what is best for their children. They have perpetuated the idea that babies "graduate" from purees to finger foods with a selection of packaged snacks and meals for toddlers. Just like I don't buy my children jarred baby food and squeeze pouches, I don't buy packaged toddler snacks and meals either. With these products, the industry is helping put young children on the processed food bandwagon so that it only seems natural to them to eat food from a box, bag, or jar. Even worse, many of these packaged products are grossly lacking in nutrition, full of sugar, and not made with real food.

Packaged Toddler Food Is Despicable—and Addicting

When you think about packaged toddler food, Gerber is the quintessential brand, with an extensive line of microwavable toddler meals, and toddler crackers, snacks, and puffs. There really isn't a more popular toddler food brand in the U.S. than Gerber, so I'm going to use it as an example.

When I first investigated Gerber's toddler products, I was pretty shocked by how long the ingredient lists were. I was even more shocked when I realized that Gerber is allowed to produce food for small children with ingredients that stimulate their taste buds to the point of addiction.

Take a look at the ingredients in a few of their toddler meals, such as their Macaroni & Cheese and Mashed Potatoes & Gravy with Roasted Chicken, and you'll find they contain additives like "autolyzed yeast extract" and "torula yeast." Instead of using monosodium glutamate (MSG), a controversial additive almost everyone is familiar with, Gerber sneaks in lesser-known additives that also contain free glutamic acid—the main component of MSG that makes food addictive. These ingredients are used solely as flavor enhancers. This is a super shady trick that allows them to essentially add MSG right under our noses to get our children hooked on processed food.

Gerber Mealtime for Toddler Mashed Potatoes & Gravy with Roasted Chicken and a side of carrots: Mashed Potatoes (Water, Potatoes, Nonfat Milk, Butter, Cream, Potassium Chloride, Salt, **Natural Flavors**, Citric Acid), Carrots, Gravy (Water, Modified Corn Starch, Maltodextrin, Chicken Broth, Wheat Flour, Chicken Fat, **Autolyzed Yeast Extract**, Dried Onion, Milk, Sodium Caseinate, Olive Oil, Potassium Chloride, Garlic Powder, Salt, Guar Gum, Xanthan Gum, Egg Yolks, Spices [Contains Celery], Caramel Color, **Natural Flavors**), Cooked Seasoned Diced Chicken Meat (Chicken Meat, Water, Corn Starch, Salt). Packed In Seasoned Water (Water, Modified Corn Starch, Sugar, Chicken Broth, Salt, Dried Onion, **Autolyzed Yeast Extract, Natural Flavor,** Lemon Juice Concentrate, Celery And Carrot Juice Concentrates).

Gerber Mealtime for Toddler Macaroni & Cheese and a side of seasoned peas & carrots: Water, Cheddar Cheese [Cultured Milk, Salt, Enzymes], Nonfat Milk, Modified Corn Starch, Cornstarch, Cream, Less Than 1% Of: Butter, Disodium Phosphate, Soy Lecithin, Salt, Potassium Chloride, **Torula Yeast, Autolyzed Yeast Extract, Natural Flavors,** Annatto and Paprika Extract Colors, Nonfat Dry Milk), Cooked Enriched Macaroni Product (Water, Wheat Semolina, Egg White, Niacin, Ferrous Sulfate, Thiamine Mononitrate, Riboflavin, Folic Acid), Water, Carrots, Peas, Squash, Less Than 1% Of: Modified Corn Starch, Chicken Broth, Dried Onion, **Autolyzed Yeast Extract, Natural Flavors,** Lemon Juice Concentrate, Salt, Celery And Carrot Juice Concentrates.

Gerber's website says they are "Offering wholesome nutrition with none of the hassle!"[12] This promise is enticing for busy parents, but the real hassle may come years down the road when your children are addicted to processed packaged foods full of hidden MSG, and haven't learned to love eating real food.

This is why I say that brands like Gerber are fundamental in getting our kids hooked on processed products from a young age—not to mention their rampant use of the mysterious additive "natural flavors," which are concoctions made in a lab to make processed food taste irresistible. These added flavors give processed food a taste that you (and your children) will never forget, and unfortunately that is a taste that isn't well replicated in real food.

Gerber is also guilty of using the risky ingredient carrageenan, a thickener and emulsifier linked to digestive problems and intestinal inflammation. It is considered by the FDA to be safe in our food, but tests have found food-grade carrageenan contaminated with up to 25 percent of "degraded carrageenan." The degraded form of carrageenan is not suitable for food, as it is classified as a "possible human carcinogen" by the International Agency for Research on Cancer. Further, when you ingest food-grade carrageenan, it can turn into the degraded version when it is exposed to stomach acid. I don't feel safe feeding my children an ingredient that's comprised of up to 25 percent carcinogens and may lead to intestinal inflammation (and maybe even cancer).

Gerber Mealtime for Toddler Pick-Ups Cheese & Spinach Ravioli: Cooked Cheese And Spinach Ravioli (Water, Whole Wheat Flour, Enriched Semolina Flour [Semolina, Niacin, Reduced Iron, Thiamin Mononitrate, Riboflavin, Folic Acid], Ricotta Cheese [Milk, Distilled Vinegar, Salt, **Carrageenan**], Eggs, Cracker Meal [Wheat Flour, Niacin, Reduced Iron Thiamine Mononitrate, Riboflavin, Folic Acid] Mozzarella Cheese Cultured Part-Skim Milk Salt, Enzymes], Spinach, Salt, Romano Cheese [Cultured Cow's Milk, Salt, Enzymes], Canola Oil, Dried Parsley), Water, Less Than 1% Of: Sugar, Cheddar Cheese [Cultured Milk, Salt Enzymes], Salt, Potassium Salt, **Autolyzed Yeast Extract**, Lemon Juice Concentrate, **Natural Flavors**.

Cheetos for Babies?

I hate to sound alarmist, but Gerber's cheddar Lil' Crunchies are nothing more than Cheetos for babies. They have very similar ingredients as Cheetos Simply Puffs, spiked with hidden MSG and natural flavor for good measure. Common sense should tell you that babies don't need Cheetos in their life, yet Gerber recommends this processed snack to babies who are only eight months old. Sheesh!

Gerber Snacks For Baby Lil' Crunchies Mild Cheddar: Whole Grain Sorghum Meal, Degermed Yellow Corn Meal, High Oleic Sunflower Oil, Cheese Seasoning (Maltodextrin, Salt, Cheddar Cheese [Cultured Milk, Salt, Enzymes], Butter Fat, **Natural Cheddar Cheese Flavor**, Annatto Extract Color, Disodium Phosphate, **Autolyzed Yeast Extract**), Calcium Carbonate, Mixed Tocopherols (To Maintain Freshness), Vitamins And Minerals: Iron (Electrolytic), Vitamin E (Alpha Tocopheryl Acetate).

Cheetos Simply Puffs: Enriched Corn Meal (Corn Meal, Ferrous Sulfate, Niacin, Thiamin Mononitrate, Riboflavin, Folic Acid), Sunflower Oil, Cheddar Cheese (Milk, Cheese Cultures, Salt, Enzymes), Whey, Maltodextrin (Made From Corn), Sea Salt, **Natural Flavors**, Sour Cream (Cultured Cream, Skim Milk), **Torula Yeast**, Lactic Acid, and Citric Acid.

Lil' Crunchies have no intrinsic nutritional value, and when babies eat ultra-processed foods like this it is reinforcing a love for crunchy, cheesy snacks that come out of a package instead of nurturing a craving for real food.

"Biscuits" Are Just Cookies

The ever-popular Arrowroot Biscuits, which Gerber calls "Your Little One's First

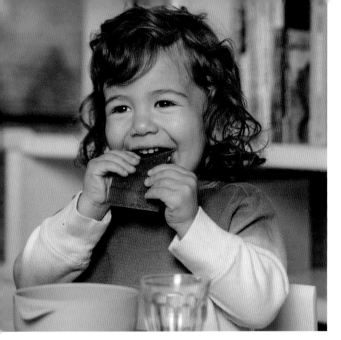

Biscuit," don't have a shred of real nutrition in them. Sure, they add some iron and vitamin E synthetically, but these cookies are primarily made with refined white flour and white sugar. One cookie boasts one gram of added sugar—and I'd bet that most babies eat several in one sitting.

You may find organic brands of arrowroot cookies with some healthier ingredients. However, these cookies will likely still be spiked with added refined sugar. Make sure to check the ingredients and remember that organic doesn't always equate to healthy ingredients.

It's no wonder kids don't like vegetables. Their taste buds are being hijacked at every meal with natural flavors, autolyzed yeast extract, and copious amounts of sugar.

Sugar, Sugar, Everywhere

You may have heard the guidelines that say adult women should eat fewer than 25 grams of added sugar per day and men should eat fewer than 38 grams of added sugar per day for good health. This is, respectively, 6 to 9 teaspoons of added sugar per day. "Added sugar" doesn't include sugar that is naturally present in whole foods like fruits and carrots. These guidelines refer to sugar that is added to processed foods, usually in the form of white sugar, cane syrup, corn syrup, and brown sugar.

Daily sugar recommendations are much stricter for young children. In fact, the American Academy of Pediatrics recommends that children under two don't consume any added sugar, and that the only sugars in their diet should be those naturally found in whole foods.[13] Yet, the Big Food industry doesn't seem to care—they still add refined sugar to virtually everything they produce. The vast majority of store-bought toddler snacks include added refined sugar, even organic brands like Plum Organics. How many toddlers eat more than one of these sugar-filled snacks a day?

Here are some common types of added refined sugar used in packaged toddler food:

- Sugar
- Cane Sugar
- Cane Syrup
- Corn Syrup
- Brown Rice Syrup
- Invert Sugar
- Evaporated Cane Invert Syrup
- Brown Sugar
- Fruit Juice Concentrate (any juice concentrate, such as apple juice concentrate)

Where's the Real Fruit?

Gerber Blueberry Puffs don't contain blueberries. These puffs are comprised of grains and white sugar that are flavored with "natural blueberry vanilla flavor" made with blueberry juice concentrate. This concoction is not similar to a real blueberry. Not even close. Adding a few drops of blueberry juice concentrate to a processed flavoring ingredient does little to improve the nutritional profile of the snack. This is just a marketing trick.

Another good example of a processed snack masquerading as real food is the ubiquitous "fruit snack." The majority of so-called fruit snacks on the market contain very little (if any) real fruit or nutrition. Annie's Organic Berry Patch Bunny Fruit Snacks are made with zero berries. Instead they use pear juice "concentrate" combined with natural flavors and refined sugar to make the gummies taste like berries—because this process is cheaper than using real berries. You may assume you're feeding your child fruit, and may believe it's a healthy snack because it is "organic"—but in reality, these snacks are heavily processed and similar to candy.

To make a concentrate, fruit puree or juice is heated and concentrated into a syrup, which is higher in sugar, lower in fiber, and lower in nutrients than whole fruit. According to Vasanti Malik, a research scientist at the Harvard T. H. Chan School of Public Health, people should view fruit concentrate as an added sugar, similar to high-fructose corn syrup.[14]

To illustrate this, one serving of Annie's Bunny Fruit Snacks (made with pear juice concentrate as the only "fruit" on the ingredient list) contains 12 grams of sugar and 0 grams of fiber. If you were to eat ½ cup real strawberries, you'd consume 4 grams of sugar with about 2 grams of fiber—and several valuable vitamins, minerals, and micronutrients. Plus, real strawberries don't come in a shiny wrapper that reinforces the idea that food comes from a package instead of from the earth. For all of these reasons, whole fruit is best. Not only is it more nutritious but eating whole fruit instead of "fruit snacks" teaches children what real food tastes like.

PACKAGED BABY FOOD & TODDLER SNACKS

Whole real food, like fruits and vegetables, should always be an option at daycares, and if it's not, I would lobby the management to start allowing it. But, if you've got no other option than providing packaged snacks for your little one, give these organic products a try. (But don't rely on them on a regular basis when you're at home and have the choice.)

- Natierra freeze-dried fruit and vegetables
- Peaceful Fruits Organic Fruit Strips
- Serenity Kids pouches (not fruit based)
- Once Upon a Farm organic baby food pouches
- Lundberg Family Farms brown rice cakes and Thin Stackers
- Lesser Evil Lil' Puffs

- That's It Organic Dried Apples
- Gaea organic olives
- Epic Salmon Smoked Maple Strip
- Amara organic baby food
- Truvani The Only Bar

A DAY IN THE LIFE OF FEEDING A TODDLER

The following is a glimpse into what feeding a toddler looks like in my home. Please note a few things:

- Like most toddlers, my children do not always finish everything on their plates. The examples outlined here are what my children start out with and what I offer to them; but they often won't eat everything, and that's okay.

- Instead of serving the entire meal at once, I usually serve the meal in courses (unless we are in a hurry to get somewhere or running late). For instance, I will offer the vegetables first. And then, I'll add in a protein. Then we'll move on to another vegetable, et cetera.

- I serve each of these meals with water.

Breakfast

Breakfast for my children is always whatever I am eating, plus a few of their favorites. I love making steel-cut oats in a crockpot overnight (on low) so it's ready to roll first thing in the morning. The whole family loves these oats. We pair them with some ground flaxseeds, cinnamon, and fruit. (Harley's favorite is pomegranate seeds and blueberries.) Another favorite is the Fast Green Waffles (page 105). I make a huge batch over the weekend, so I can thaw them out in our mini-oven (300°F for 6 minutes) on busy mornings.

Snack 1

We usually offer a midmorning snack that is leftover breakfast. On many days, Finley is so full from nursing first thing in the morning that he won't eat much of his breakfast. Instead of throwing away his food, we'll offer it to him again as a snack and then usually thaw out one buckwheat pancake. I make a bunch and freeze them (separated by parchment paper). I use Arrowhead Mills Organic Buckwheat Pancake & Waffle Mix, but add an extra egg and one mashed banana to the mixture instead of honey. I serve it without syrup.

Lunch

Typically, we serve one steamed vegetable, some type of bean, and Finley's favorite pasta and some fruit. If he is still hungry, he'll dig out of my salad bowl till he's satisfied. If I am drinking a smoothie for lunch, he loves to take a few sips, or I'll offer him some hummus and carrots.

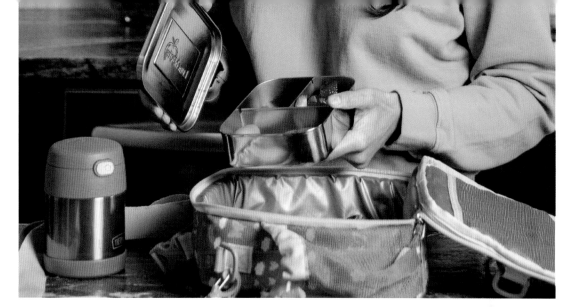

Snack 2

This happens after he wakes up from his nap. Finley likes to nurse and then have some Crispy Ranch Chickpeas (page 160) plus some fruit (watermelon balls are the current favorite). Finley loves olives and organic dried fruit without added sugar and will ask for most snacks by name!

Are your kids always helping themselves to a snack? Finley got so used to following his big sister into the pantry that we had to add a lock to the pantry door, because he was starting to snack at all times of the day. Just adding the lock lets him know there is a boundary with snacks, and it has reduced the number of times he asks for a snack during the day. Mealtimes can often be sabotaged if my kids snack too much.

Dinner

We almost always eat the exact same dinner as our children. On this day, I made wild salmon, quinoa, sautéed purple cabbage, and sautéed kale in olive oil for us all, and the kids had some frozen peas, raspberries, and pomegranate seeds for dessert.

PACKING SCHOOL LUNCHES

I used to eat the same thing for lunch every day at school. Both of my parents worked full-time, so I sometimes had to make my lunch myself. I'd fill a paper bag with a peanut butter-and-jelly sandwich, an apple, and a bag of Frito chips. This was my go-to lunch every day of the week, and it never included any green vegetables. My kids are not going to know what that was like. As you know, my top priority is making sure my family eats well, so packing my kids a healthy lunch with vegetables is not negotiable. You won't find Goldfish crackers, Lunchables, and processed meat in their lunch boxes. Their lunches may be a little different than those of the other kids at school, but since it's the same food that they love to eat at home, it's comforting nonetheless.

I encourage you to make packing lunches for your kids one of your top priorities too, because it is so rewarding—and it's imperative for helping them develop a love for real food.

I've noticed that my daughter doesn't eat well in the distracted environment at school. That's why in the morning, before I take her to school, I offer her a hearty breakfast full of vegetables, good whole grains like steel-cut oats, and healthy fats like flaxseed, along with fruit. For her lunch, I like to pack at least two different vegetables and one fruit, one carb, one protein, and typically one fun treat. One of these items is served hot or warm, packed in a thermos.

Mix-and-Match Lunch Ideas Chart

Below you'll find some ideas for each category of food discussed above. Of course, these aren't all the good options available—they're just a starting point based on what I pack for my child. All items listed below are organic.

VEGETABLES (Choose Two)

Generally vegetables are steamed or roasted, served either warm or cold.
Older children can be given raw veggie sticks with dip.

Roasted Cauliflower (page 260)
Carrots
Bell Pepper Slices (red, yellow, or orange)
Broccoli
Vegetable Soup
Snap Peas

Peas
Green Beans
Zucchini
Salad (leafy greens with dressing on the side)
Fresh Cherry Tomato & Cucumber Salad (page 184)

FRUIT (Choose One)

Chia Seed Fruit Salad (page 102)
Apple Slices
Strawberries
Blueberries
Bananas
Avocados
Oranges
Melons (cubed)

CARB/STARCH (Choose One)

Sprouted Rice
Rice & Beans
Quinoa
Lentil Pasta
Beet Chips
Whole Grain or Rice Crackers
Sweet Potato (roasted, mashed, or diced)
Sprouted Pita
Sprouted Tortilla

PROTEIN (Choose One)

Lentil Pasta (serves as both starch and protein)
Pinto Beans (page 259)
Shredded Chicken
Grilled Diced Chicken
Chicken Wings
Ground Turkey
Chicken Sausage
Goat Cheese Mozzarella or Cheddar Slices
Salmon Balls (page 156)
Teriyaki Pork Tenderloin (page 209)

TREAT (Choose One)

Carrot Cake Muffin (page 101)
Real Food Fruit Leather (page 180)
Dried Cherries
Chocolate-Covered Goji Berries
Dried Cranberries
Homemade Fig Newtons (Recipe in *Food Babe Kitchen* or at foodbabe.com/resources)

Sometimes a few of these items will be prepared together into one dish. To give you an idea of how I put it all together, let me show you the lunches I packed for Harley's first week of school.

Real-Life Lunch Box Examples

Day 1 – Cauliflower and Carrots (roasted with olive oil, sea salt, pepper, and paprika), Apple Slices, Grilled Chicken, Dried Cherries

Day 2 – Rice and Beans, Orange Bell Pepper Slices, Cheese Slices, Rustic Bakery Crackers, Apple Slices, Dried Cherries, and Beet Chips

Day 3 – Lentil Pasta (made with tomato sauce and freshly grated Parmesan), Cucumbers, Strawberries, Date Stuffed with Almond Butter (if your school is nut free, you can use sunflower butter)

Day 4 – Mediterranean Chickpea Salad, Blueberries, Carrot Cake Muffins, Real Food Fruit Leather

Day 5 – Chicken Wings with Roasted Brussels Sprouts, Pear Tomatoes, Real Food Fruit Leather

As you can see, I didn't pack the exact same thing each day, but I repeated some items. I also included several options of vegetables. When it comes to packing lunch, variety is key! This is very important if you have a picky eater, as exposing your child to a variety of foods will help them become more adventurous.

Bookmark These Recipes!

Here you will find a few of my picks for easy recipes that are perfect for lunch boxes and thermoses. You can prepare a few of these items ahead of time and store them in the fridge for the week. You can then round out this list with some carefully selected organic store-bought items (such as sprouted pita bread), fruits, and vegetables.

- Ultimate Veggie Pasta Salad (page 200)
- Carrot Lentil Soup (page 196)
- Food Babe's Favorite Green Beans (page 248)
- Roasted Cauliflower (page 260)
- Easy Parmesan Broccoli (page 256)
- Easy Chicken Quinoa Chili (page 223)
- Turkey Lettuce Wraps (page 206)
- Meatball Skewers (page 220)
- Teriyaki Pork Tenderloin (page 209)
- No Fuss Ginger Chicken Stir-Fry with Broccoli (page 235)
- Carrot Cake Muffins (page 101)
- Better-for-You "Rice Krispies" Treats (page 273)
- Real Food Fruit Leather (page 180)

Guidelines for Packing a Healthy Lunch Your Child Will Love

Include dips! Children love to dip their food. Raw veggies can be especially boring

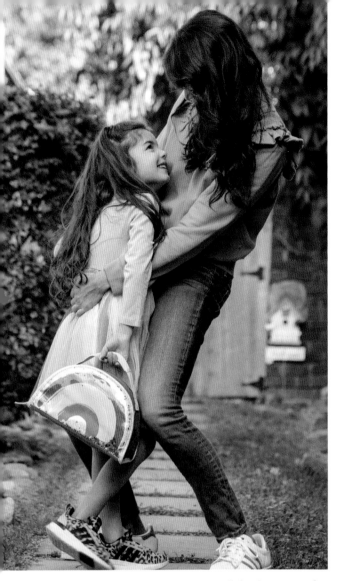

Even roasting cauliflower is fairly quick and something you can do ahead of time and store in the fridge until it's time to pack.

Include fun touches when you have time. Write your child a note or draw them a funny picture and stick it inside their lunch box. You can find cute reusable toothpicks with soft edges that are decorated with characters that they love; stick the toothpicks into cheese cubes or fruit slices.

Don't pack exactly the same thing every day in a row. This is pretty obvious, but your child will get bored with their food if they see the same thing every day. Mix it up, without completely changing their lunch each day. For example, you might steam green beans and pack them in their lunch on Monday, Wednesday, and Friday. On other days, try to pack a different vegetable. The following week, choose different vegetables and rotate.

Offer variety. Stick to the ideas chart and the categories provided and you'll be all set! Give your child a few options in their lunch to choose from. For instance add a couple different vegetables and a piece of fruit, so hopefully they will eat at least one of them during lunch.

Include their favorites and familiar foods. You don't want your child to open their lunch box and be stunned by an array of foods that they don't normally eat. It's best to introduce a new food at home several times first before you pack it in their

unless you have dips. You'll find recipes for my favorite dips on pages 170–175.

Keep it simple. You don't have to make everything from scratch. You also don't need to cut everything into a flower or Instagram-worthy robot shape. Fun is fun if you have time, but I keep it simple. Choose one to two items from each category in the ideas chart (page 18). Many of the items won't require too much work, such as slicing strawberries.

lunch box. Always include at least one favorite healthy food that you know they'll eat.

After-school snack. Allow your child to finish their lunch after school. If they don't finish their lunch at school, the leftovers can make a great after-school snack. Harley often wants to eat the rest of her lunch after school because she doesn't have enough time to eat it all during her lunch hour.

We've learned why most children hate vegetables and why it's a good idea to get them started with real food right off the bat. The best way to do this is to consistently provide whole foods (vegetables, fruits, grains, etc) to your children and minimize their exposure to processed food as much as possible. This will put them on the road to loving real food, which is one of the greatest gifts your can give your children. In the next chapter, we'll take a virtual trip to the grocery store, where I'll show you how to avoid misleading labels on packages and how to choose the healthiest snacks and drinks for your family.

How to Pack a Hot Lunch (That Stays Hot!)

When Harley started having lunch at school (around her kindergarten year), I really wanted to make sure she had something warm in her lunch each day. I love to pack her pasta dishes, rice and beans, and roasted vegetables. This way she has comforting hot food from home to eat if she's feeling cold or if the air-conditioning is on too high (which is common in many places). Keeping her food hot until lunchtime can be a challenge, especially since her school is required by law to store each child's lunch box in the fridge. Thankfully, though, this rule doesn't apply to insulated thermoses.

The first thermos I tried kept Harley's food hot but wasn't easy for her to open on her own. I wanted her to be independent, so then I tried one with an easy snap lid—but that one didn't keep her food hot. I eventually picked my battle. I gave her the harder-to-open thermos, and she asks for help when she needs it. So you may have to experiment before you find a thermos that works for you and your child.

Here are a few more tricks to ease the process and keep your child's food warm for hours:

- Prep all the cold lunch items the night before and stash them in the fridge. That way the only thing left to do in the morning is heat up the hot food and pack it.

- While you're in the kitchen preparing breakfast, this is a great time to multitask. Heat up your child's hot lunch item on the stove or in the oven at the same time.

- Preheat your thermos by pouring boiling hot water into it. Dump out the water before adding the hot food.

- Make sure that you don't pack the hot food until the last minute before your child needs to leave for school. You want it in the thermos for the least amount of time, so it stays hot longer.

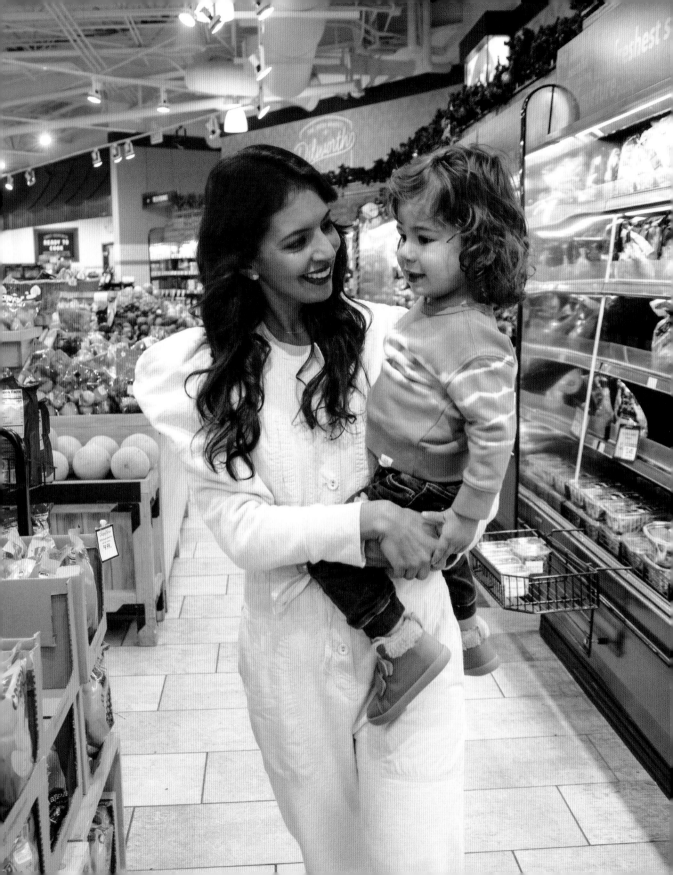

chapter 2

BUYING THE HEALTHIEST FOOD FOR YOUR FAMILY

From the moment you walk into your average supermarket, you are being targeted. Big Food manufacturers spend vast resources on marketing and store placements to make sure that you (and your children) see what they want you to see, and feel compelled to buy their latest creations.[1] If you've ever heard the advice to "shop the perimeter" in the store and avoid the center aisles, this is pretty good advice. That's because the perimeter of the store is typically where you will find the real food. That being said, this is much easier said than done. It can be difficult to resist the colorful displays of packaged products, especially when you've got little ones in tow!

Let's delve into how to spot dirty tricks designed to persuade you to buy unhealthy processed food. Then we'll take a look at the good, the bad, and the ugly in the grocery store, so that next time you are shopping for food you won't get suckered into buying junk food disguised as health food.

RIDICULOUS KID-FOOD MARKETING

Right on the can of SpaghettiOs it claims the product is a "Healthy Kids Entree" that provides four essential nutrients and 20 percent of daily vegetables. They go on to say that one cup of canned pasta equals half a cup of vegetables. Campbell's wants parents to believe that SpaghettiOs are a great source of vegetables for your child. They've got to be kidding, right?

Where are the vegetables?

SpaghettiOs Ingredients: Water, Tomato Puree (Water, Tomato Paste), Enriched Pasta (Wheat Flour, Niacin, Ferrous Sulfate, Thiamine

Mononitrate, Riboflavin, Folic Acid), High-Fructose Corn Syrup. Contains Less Than 2% Of: Salt, Enzyme Modified Cheddar Cheese (Cheddar Cheese [Cultured Milk, Salt, Enzymes, Calcium Chloride], Water, Disodium Phosphate, Enzymes), Vegetable Oil (Corn, Canola, and/or Soybean), Enzyme Modified Butter, Beta Carotene For Color, Citric Acid, Paprika Extract, Skim Milk, Natural Flavoring.

This is what I call ridiculous kid-food marketing. Those "vegetables" in a can of SpaghettiOs are in the form of tomato paste (tomatoes cooked for hours and strained), which is then mixed with high-fructose corn syrup and flavors to make it taste more appealing to children. That's about as ridiculous as calling Heinz ketchup a vegetable!

Unfortunately, thousands of parents believe that SpaghettiOs are a healthy dinner for their kids in a pinch. The Big Food industry has very deep pockets. They have the means to keep marketing their lies and pushing toxic products on families. This is why it's important to read the ingredient lists instead of the marketing slogans on the package.

Let's look at some other ridiculous marketing examples. Kellogg's says their Strawberry Nutri-Grain Bites are made with real fruit, 8 grams of whole grains, and no artificial flavors. Sounds pretty good, right?

Upon closer inspection you'll find that the "real fruit" strawberry filling is mostly made from inverted sugar and fructose that has been flavored and colored to taste and look like strawberries. This sugary filling includes thickeners such as cellulose gel and cellulose gum, which are linked in

some research to weight gain, inflammation, and digestive problems. They do add some processed "strawberry puree concentrate," which allows them to use the "real fruit" claim on the package—but I think you'd agree that the result isn't anywhere close to real strawberries.

Hi-C Orange Lavaburst drinks claim to give your child a full day's supply of vitamin C. Supposedly, they are "made with real fruit juice," with "the great taste your kids will love." That last part may be true, but I guarantee that you won't love knowing that each box of Hi-C consists mostly of high-fructose corn syrup and water. These little sugar bombs are also filled with two artificial sweeteners: sucralose and acesulfame potassium. These ingredients are both linked in some animal research to cancer,[2] and sucralose is specifically linked to leukemia.[3] There are surely better sources of vitamin C for our children!

The next time you see claims like the ones listed below, make sure you take a very close look at the ingredient label:

- "**Good Source of Calcium and Vitamin D**": Does this product naturally contain the nutrients claimed or is it a refined product that has synthetic nutrients added back in?

- "**No Artificial Flavors**": Does this product contain natural flavors instead? Natural flavors are not very different from artificial flavors, so this isn't a real improvement.

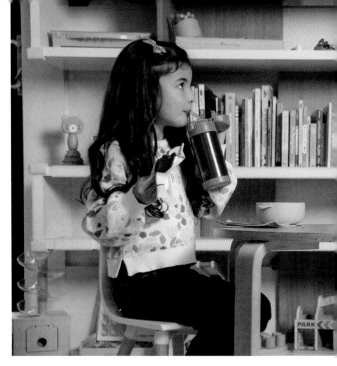

- **"No Artificial Colors"**: It's great that this product isn't artificially dyed—but why would it need any colors in the first place? Usually products that have colors added (even natural colors) are processed products. Ask yourself if this product is real food.

- **"No High-Fructose Corn Syrup"**: What is this product sweetened with instead? Does this product still contain corn syrup or white sugar? Does it contain artificial sweeteners like sucralose or acesulfame potassium?

- **"Made with Whole Grains"**: Does this product still contain refined grains? What about refined oils or sugar?

This is not the only way the processed food industry will swindle you into buying their products. It really gets me when I see popular cartoon characters on products that have horrible ingredients for kids. This is the lowest of the low when it comes to Big Food marketing tricks. I stopped dead in my tracks when I first saw Kellogg's Baby Shark Cereal, a character that my daughter loved at the time. I knew that if she saw this in the store, she would relentlessly beg for a box—but there is no way I would agree to buy her a product full of artificial colors linked to hyperactivity and immune system disruption, not to mention all the sugar and refined ingredients this product contains. A few years later, I was astonished again when I saw that Pepperidge Farm came out with Goldfish crackers shaped like Disney princesses Jasmine, Moana, and Cinderella (packaged with cute little pink Goldfish). My daughter would go bonkers for these! But I'm not interested in supporting companies who market products for children that are primarily filled with refined and processed ingredients. I'll delve into specifically why I don't buy Goldfish crackers later in this chapter. There are much healthier options out there in the market today. And although other options aren't shaped into Disney characters, at least they are better for her body.

Don't be swindled by Big Food marketing lies and tricks! Remember that you have the power in your own hands. Read the ingredient label on all of the products you buy for your kids, and if they aren't made with real ingredients (like what you'd find in your own kitchen), seek out better alternatives or make a homemade version yourself.

Fighting Back against Kellogg's: The Dirtiest Marketing Trick in the Book!

When I first saw Kellogg's Baby Shark Cereal my heart sank. My daughter was two years old at the time and absolutely loved the "Baby Shark" song and dance. I knew when she saw Baby Shark on a box of cereal at the store, she'd beg me to buy it. But I didn't even need to look at the ingredients to know that this wouldn't be something I'd want to buy for her. However, I decided to read the ingredients anyway, and what I saw made me so angry: the cereal was packed with artificial colors, which are linked to immune system dysfunction and hyperactivity in children. I got angrier still when I remembered that Kellogg's announced plans in 2015[4] to remove artificial colors and artificial flavors from all of their cereals by the end of 2018. But they never did. Kellogg's continues to sell several cereals that contain artificial colors and flavors. Kellogg's is saying one thing but doing another. Where is their integrity? Meanwhile, Kellogg's sells cereals with safer ingredients in other countries. In Europe and Australia, Kellogg's takes artificial colors and the risky preservative BHT out of their cereals completely. Why not here too?

I had to do something. I wanted to hold Kellogg's accountable. In September 2019 I launched a petition asking Kellogg's to keep their word and remove all artificial colors, artificial flavors, and BHT from their cereals. The Food Babe Army went wild sharing this petition; we collected over 16,000 signatures in the first 24 hours. I made a live TV appearance to really get Kellogg's attention. I wanted everyone to know about this petition and how we could band together to make a change. This is when we received an official response from Kellogg's, which basically told us to pound sand.

Kellogg's wrote, "Ultimately, we will not sacrifice the great taste and quality consumers expect from their favorite Kellogg's products."

I'd venture a guess that most people buying Baby Shark Cereal wouldn't care about the "great taste and quality" if they knew how these artificial ingredients could be affecting their children's bodies. Kellogg's already knows how to make Froot Loops without artificial colors, as they have done so in other markets—and they can feasibly do the same with all their children's cereals.

We kept pushing. Within a few months we had gathered over 50,000 signatures. It was now time to box them up and take the signed petitions to Kellogg's headquarters in Battle Creek, Michigan, to request a meeting. Right as I was getting ready to book a flight and make this happen, the unexpected happened. The world came to a screeching halt when Covid hit, and I knew it would be several months (if not longer) before I'd be able to travel or meet with their executives. What was I going to do now?

I came up with a plan. I figured out how to get authorized by a shareholder to act as their representative at Kellogg's virtual shareholder's meeting in Spring 2020. During the early part of the pandemic, this was my only way to be personally heard by Kellogg's CEO and executives. I was only permitted to submit written questions, and there was the risk that the moderator would ignore my questions. Although I submitted several, only one of my questions was read and answered during the meeting.[5] I asked, "What is your current position on removing artificial colors from all your cereals, such as Froot Loops and Apple Jacks?"

Steven Cahillane, the CEO of Kellogg's responded: "We have made tremendous progress in removing artificial ingredients from all of our products including our ready-to-eat cereal products. Where we will not make compromise is around taste and enjoyment, and so, to the extent that we can continue to make progress and delight consumers with non-compromising foods, that's our north star."

Kellogg's is sacrificing children's health to "delight consumers." Maddening, isn't it? That is why I have refused to give up. Kellogg's still has not made the changes and is still creating new cereals with artificial ingredients for our kids.

I'm confident that Kellogg's will eventually change, but it will take all of us to demand it. When we petitioned Kraft in 2013, and I arrived uninvited at their headquarters with thousands of petition signatures asking them to remove artificial colors from their Mac & Cheese, they reluctantly agreed to meet with me. I'll never forget what they told me: "We'll have to agree to disagree." They went on to say that their customers like Kraft Mac & Cheese just the way it was, with artificial colors. Well, guess what happened next?! Kraft removed the artificial colors after all, in 2016. We influenced Kraft to change their iconic Mac & Cheese, and I know in my heart that we can influence Kellogg's to do the same with Froot Loops, Apple Jacks, Baby Shark, and all their cereals.

If you're a concerned parent who'd like to add your name to the petition, you can do so here:
FoodBabe.com/BabyShark

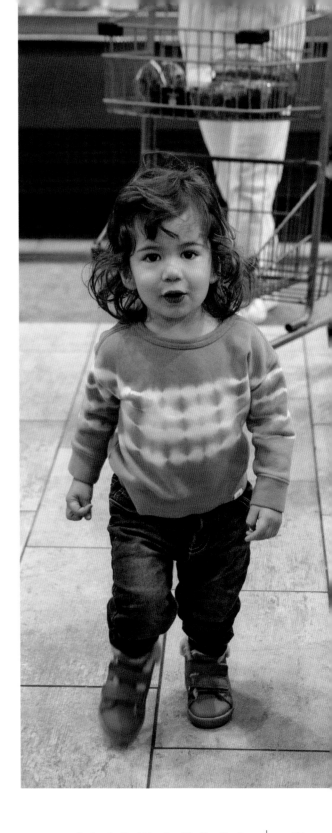

38 Percent of Children Believe Chicken Nuggets Come from Plants

A 2021 study published in the *Journal of Environmental Psychology* found that 38 percent of American children believe that chicken nuggets come from plants.[6] Researchers asked 4- to 7-year-old children from the United States to identify different foods and determine whether each one was plant based or animal based. In the study, almost all the foods were incorrectly identified by 30 percent of the children (with the exception of milk), including french fries—which 47 percent of the children believed came from an animal.

While the results of this study are disheartening, they're not surprising: If children are getting the majority of their food from a box, jar, squeeze pack, or fast-food window, I can see how they are confused about where our food comes from. For example, eating slices of fresh banana is not the same experience as sucking mashed banana from a plastic pouch, or off a spoon from a jar. When your child eats a real banana, they can smell it and mash it between their fingers (and perhaps even smoosh it into their hair). This is a valuable learning experience for your child, which helps them understand what real food smells, looks, and tastes like. Later on, when your child sees bananas in the produce section at the store, they will start to associate them with the bananas they've been eating at home. If they've been solely eating bananas from a jar of baby food, they may not make this connection.

Try these tips to help your children learn about where our food comes from:

- Take them with you to the farmer's market or grocery store. Show them the fresh produce and talk to them about how it is grown. Let them feel, smell, and add the fresh produce to your basket or cart.

- Let them watch you in the kitchen as you wash produce and chop vegetables. Talk to them about each ingredient and where it comes from. For example, you can say, "These are orange carrots that are grown in the ground. They are crunchy and sweet."

- Start a small garden at home, even if it's just a simple herb garden, and let them help you nurture the plants and enjoy what they produce. Not in a million years could I predict my daughter's favorite vegetable would be bok choy if we hadn't first grown it in our front porch planters one summer. She loved picking the bok choy with her dad; and when he cooked it with garlic, olive oil, and lemon, she just couldn't get enough. The whole process of planting the seeds, watching the plant grow, and getting to eat it helped her love this vegetable.

- When they're old enough, serve your babies fresh fruits and vegetables and let them play with it (even if they don't eat it at first). This will help them learn about all the different tastes, smells, and textures that are abundant in nature. Good ones to start with are avocados, steamed broccoli, green beans, bananas, and watermelon slices.

- Read children's books about food and teach them where different fruits and vegetables are grown and where animal products come from. One of my favorite children's books is called *Buddies in the Belly*; it teaches kids all about the beneficial bacteria in various fruits and vegetables and how they help you stay healthy.

THE TERRIBLE 10: THE WORST INGREDIENTS IN CHILDREN'S FOOD

To help you make informed decisions at the grocery store, I put together this list of the 10 most harmful ingredients that are commonly found in children's food. I explain why to avoid them, which products contain them, and what to look for on the label. I'd love to say that these ingredients are easy to avoid, but that's simply not the truth. Pick up almost any popular children's product out there and it's very likely that it contains at least one (or more) of the following:

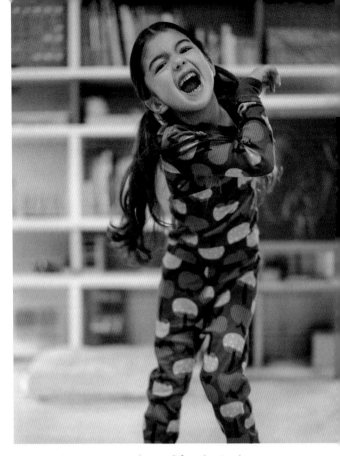

1. Refined Sugar
2. MSG and "Hidden MSG" Additives
3. Growth Hormones
4. Antibiotics
5. Pesticides
6. Artificial Dyes and Colors
7. Refined Flour and Enriched Flour
8. Preservatives
9. Natural and Artificial Flavors
10. Heavy Metals

Let's break each of these down into more detail.

1. Refined Sugar

Children (and adults alike) have no nutritional need for refined sugar, yet you'll find it added to most packaged foods. Pediatric experts say that children under the age of two shouldn't be eating refined sugar at all, and that the only sugar in their diet should come naturally from whole foods (such as the sugar in a banana).

Found in: SpaghettiOs, Lovebird Honey Cereal, Cheerios, Mott's Original Applesauce, Fruit by the Foot, Welch's Fruit Snacks, Fruit Gushers, Chef Boyardee Beef Ravioli, Gerber Arrowroot Biscuits, Gerber Toddler Meals, Plum Organics Mighty Snack Bars, Gerber Grain & Grow Puffs, Beech-Nut Breakfast Pouches, LaraBar Bakes Bars, Nature's Bakery Fig Bar, Quaker Flavored Instant Oatmeal Packets.

On the label: sugar, cane sugar, brown rice syrup, evaporated cane syrup, brown sugar syrup, corn syrup, high-fructose corn syrup, and juice concentrates.

2. MSG and "Hidden MSG" Additives

Food companies use MSG and similar additives to engineer their food to taste irresistible and memorable so you eat more. This is why MSG is also linked to obesity—it causes food to taste better than it should, increasing addictive eating habits. In fact, MSG is often used in animal studies to make rats obese. MSG is listed as "monosodium glutamate" on the label; however, most brands that sell children's food sneak in other additives—such as yeast extract and hydrolyzed proteins—that contain "free glutamic acid," which is the main component of MSG. MSG is also an excitotoxin that can excite brain cells to death[7] and cause adverse reactions in some people, including skin rashes, itching, hives, nausea, vomiting, migraine headaches, asthma, heart irregularities, depression, and even seizures.[8]

Found in: Quaker Cheddar Rice Crisps, Goldfish crackers, SpaghettiOs, Yummy Dino Buddies Chicken Nuggets, Kid Cuisine Chicken Breast Nuggets, Gerber Toddler Meals, Gerber Pick-Ups, Bagel Bites, Chick-fil-A Nuggets, McDonald's McNuggets.

On the label: monosodium glutamate, autolyzed yeast extract, yeast extract, hydrolyzed soy protein, and torula yeast.

3. Growth Hormones

Cows raised for food or dairy in the United States are often given steroids, growth hormones, and drugs. These drugs are certainly unhealthy for the animals, and eating meat raised on hormones may increase the risk of diseases in humans as well, including cancer and premature puberty in children. Some conventional dairies inject their cows with synthetic hormones to increase milk production, despite evidence that it may lead to higher levels of the cancer-causing hormone IGF-1.[9]

Found in: Beef and dairy products that are not organic are at risk.

On the label: If hormones are used, it won't be listed on the package. Products that display the USDA Organic seal cannot contain added hormones. Beware that some packages state the meat has "No Added Hormones," but the animals may still have been given antibiotics or other drugs if the package doesn't indicate otherwise.

4. Antibiotics

National surveys have been done showing antibiotic residues in meats, milk, and in some cities, drinking water.[10] That means even if you avoid unnecessary antibiotics from your doctor, you could be getting them from the grocery store and faucet. The majority of antibiotics in the U.S. are fed to farm animals at constant low levels to fatten them up on less food. They're also used to prevent illnesses on factory farms. This saves the meat industry money, but it is causing a major human health crisis. Many experts agree that the overuse and misuse of antibiotics in food animals is a major source of the antibiotic-resistant bacteria that are affecting humans and leading to infections that are difficult to treat and sometimes impossible to cure. Thousands of Americans die from antibiotic-resistant bacterial infections every year, and these infections are on the rise.[11] Antibiotics kill off healthy bacteria in the gut and beneficial bugs called probiotics that influence how we absorb nutrients, burn off calories, and stay lean.

Found in: Any conventional animal product (meat, dairy, eggs) that isn't organic or doesn't carry the "Raised without Antibiotics" label. Keep this in mind when purchasing any packaged food that has animal products as an ingredient and when dining in restaurants that don't have antibiotic-free policies in place.

On the label: If antibiotics were used, that won't be listed on the package. Look for "Raised without Antibiotics" or the USDA Certified Organic seal.

5. Pesticides

Pesticides are sprayed on fruits, vegetables, grains, nuts, and seeds—virtually everything grown in nature—and they're among the most toxic substances on Earth, doing untold damage to our bodies. For one thing, they imitate estrogen (a fat-forming hormone) and disrupt thyroid function—two side effects that encourage weight gain.[12] Studies have also linked pesticide exposure to increased risk of cancer.[13] One of the most widely used herbicides is glyphosate, commonly known as Roundup. This chemical is used on genetically engineered (GMO) crops that were designed to be resistant to it, but it's also used on some non-GMO crops (oats and wheat, for example) as a drying agent. Although glyphosate has been linked to cancer[14] and other diseases, it is still widely used in the U.S.

Found in: Conventional (non-organic) produce is most likely to be contaminated with pesticides even if it is non-GMO. Also avoid common GMO foods like corn, soy, canola, sugar beets, cottonseed, papaya, zucchini, and squash, unless they are organic. Always wash your produce well, but be aware that many pesticides used are systemic, which means they infiltrate the inside of the produce and cannot be washed off.

On the label: This is a contaminate, so pesticides won't be listed on the package; however, USDA Certified Organic food is less likely to be contaminated. Use EWG's Dirty Dozen guide to determine which produce is the least contaminated with pesticides if an organic option is not available.

6. Artificial Dyes and Colors

Children in particular tend to eat with their eyes first, and food manufacturers capitalize on this. Dyed foods trick your kids by making processed food look more fun and appealing than real food. Artificial food dyes are linked to hyperactivity in children, asthma, allergies, and skin issues, and they are known to disrupt the immune system.[15] They are banned in certain countries and require a warning label in Europe,[16] which is why you'll rarely see them when traveling overseas. Titanium dioxide is used as a whitening agent in some U.S.-produced foods, even though it was banned in Europe after it was found to be potentially genotoxic.[17]

Found in: Kellogg's Unicorn Waffles, Pop Tarts, Fruit by the Foot, Welch's Fruit Snacks, Fruit Gushers, Pedialyte, SunnyD, Kool-Aid Bursts, PediaSure Grow & Gain Chocolate, Post Honeycomb Cereal, Skittles, Trix, Froot Loops.

On the label: Yellow 5, Yellow 6, Red 40, Red 3, Blue 1, titanium dioxide, and caramel color are the most common dyes found in processed food in the United States.

7. Refined Flour and/or Enriched Flour

A flour that is refined has been stripped of its nutrients and fiber, leaving behind a powdery product devoid of any life. It's dead food. Refined flour can be treated with dozens of different chemicals approved by the FDA before it ends up in our food—including chemical bleach! The flour is treated with chlorine dioxide, which leeches out vitamin E. Often, manufacturers "enrich" this dead flour by adding synthetic nutrients back into the product (niacin, reduced iron, thiamine mononitrate, riboflavin, folic acid) that are not from nature. Consuming this type of flour raises your blood sugar quickly, potentially leading to weight gain, cardiovascular disease, and type 2 diabetes. It's similar to eating refined sugar!

Found in: Goldfish crackers, Annie's Organic Cheddar Bunnies, SpaghettiOs, Chef Boyardee Beef Ravioli, Gerber Arrowroot Biscuits, Beech-Nut Mini Waffles, Honey Maid Graham Crackers, Rold Gold Tiny Pretzel Twists, Eggo Waffles, Wendy's Jr. cheeseburger, McDonald's cheeseburger, Subway sandwiches.

On the label: wheat flour, enriched flour, bleached enriched flour, unbleached wheat flour.

8. Preservatives

Preservatives increase the shelf life of packaged foods, but may have the opposite effect on our own life. The cumulative effect of consuming various preservatives has not been studied long term on humans, and many preservatives contain potential cancer-causing compounds and endocrine disruptors.[18] Among the worst of these preservatives are nitrates, used in processed meats to prevent bacterial growth and maintain the color of the meat. Toxic to the brain, nitrates are linked to Alzheimer's disease[19] and many types of cancer.[20] Then we have BHA and BHT, which are heavily restricted preservatives in other countries but widely used in the United States. These have produced cancers in animal studies, and even our own Department of Health and Human Services classifies BHA as "reasonably anticipated to be a human carcinogen"[21]—but the FDA still allows it in our food. Citric acid (made from GMO black mold) and ascorbic acid (synthetic vitamin C) are often added to baby food and pouches. These preservatives both make the food more acidic and can lead to inflammation.[22]

Found in: Fruit by the Foot, Kraft Mac & Cheese, Totino's Pizza Rolls, Gerber fruit & veggie pouches, SunnyD, Kool-Aid Bursts, Foster Farms Mini Corn Dogs, Bagel Bites, Wendy's Jr. cheeseburger, McDonald's cheeseburger, Subway sandwiches.

On the label: sodium nitrate, sodium nitrite, BHA, BHT, citric acid, ascorbic acid (preservative), potassium sorbate, sodium benzoate, sodium phosphate, calcium propionate, and TBHQ.

9. Natural Flavors and Artificial Flavors

The only difference between natural and artificial flavors is that natural flavors are derived from natural substances—plants or animals. Which sounds nice, until you realize that this includes beaver anal glands which are sometimes used to make vanilla flavoring! Each natural flavor may also contain up to 100 ingredients, including sodium benzoate, glycerin, potassium sorbate, and propylene glycol (none of which are labeled). Ultimately, these are proprietary mixtures that make food taste irresistible so that you keep coming back for more, very similar to MSG. This helps your child get hooked on processed unhealthy foods![23]

Found in: Annie's Organic Bunny Grahams, Baby Shark Macaroni & Cheese, Tyson Chicken Nuggets, Gerber Arrowroot Biscuits, Plum Organics Teensy Snacks, Baby Mum-Mum Banana Teething Wafers, Gerber Grain & Grow Puffs, Mott's Mighty Flying Fruit Punch, Barnum's Original Animal Crackers, Hippeas Chickpea Puffs, Smartfood White Cheddar Popcorn, Pirate's Booty, Nature's Bakery Fig Bar, MadeGood Granola Bars.

On the label: natural flavor, artificial flavor, organic natural flavor. Organic natural flavors won't contain synthetic additives, but they are still not considered real food, added for the same reasons that other natural flavors are used.

10. Heavy Metals

Heavy metals like aluminum, lead, mercury, and arsenic have reached our food through polluted soils and water and in processing facilities. Some types of food are more likely to be contaminated than others, due to the conditions in which they are grown, packaged, or processed. Heavy metals can be especially dangerous for babies and young children, as their brains and bodies are still developing. They are particularly toxic to brain cells. Repeated exposure to heavy metals is linked to problems with learning, cognition, and behavior. These metals accumulate in the body, increasing the risk of permanent damage with each exposure. (For a detailed explanation, see pages 7–9.)

Found in: Rice-based ingredients (brown rice, white rice, brown rice syrup, etc.) or juice concentrates such as apple juice concentrate are most likely to be contaminated with heavy metals. Products would include rice cereal, teething biscuits, puffs, and baby food and squeeze pouches made with rice or juice concentrates.

On the label: This is a naturally occurring contaminate, so it won't be listed on the label.

Now, let's discuss one of the sneakiest products in your child's diet that may not be on your radar, but that they're consuming every day: beverages!

BEST AND WORST BEVERAGES FOR KIDS: RANKED!

Pay close attention to the beverages you offer your child. Studies show that the primary source of sugar in a child's diet comes from what they drink. This is no surprise when you consider that there is an entire aisle at your local supermarket filled with sugary sodas, juice boxes, and sports drinks. One can of soda typically has over 10 teaspoons of sugar in it. This alone greatly exceeds the amount of sugar experts say children should have in a day, which is no more than 6 teaspoons of sugar for children over the age of two.[24] Too much sugar in your child's diet puts them at a much greater risk of obesity, type 2 diabetes, cancer, and other diseases. Other drinks marketed to children are oftentimes just as unhealthy and sugary as soda. Some are even promoted as good options for kids and served at schools. For example, most "100% juice" boxes are concealed sugar bombs in your child's diet. That's because they are made from reconstituted juice "concentrates," which are not the same as fresh pressed juice. To make a concentrate, juice is reduced to a syrup, essentially becoming a refined sugar. During the concentration process, natural nutrients and flavors are lost, so they add those back in artificially. The juice is often heated up to be pasteurized, which also denatures enzymes and destroys nutrients. This is a far cry from a cold-pressed orange juice, which still has a large amount of natural sugar, but its nutrients and enzymes are intact.

I offer my children just a few drink options. We serve filtered water with everything. This is the main thing that we drink as a family. Occasionally, we'll enjoy organic coconut or almond milk, mint tea, kombucha, or raw coconut water. My husband likes to drink cold-pressed orange juice, so sometimes if my daughter sees him drinking it, she'll want some. I'll pour her a little in a glass mixed with filtered water. She doesn't know the difference.

To help you sort out the best drinks for your children, I developed a ranking chart. You'll find four categories: (1) Worst Drinks for Kids, (2) Not-Much-Better Drinks for Kids, (3) Still-Not-the-Best Drinks for Kids, and (4) Best Drinks for Kids. If you are buying any of the low-ranking drinks, I don't want you to feel bad. Remember, the Big Food industry is spending millions of dollars on advertising to sell these drinks to you and your children. They know how to push your buttons. Take this ranking chart as empowering advice. Now that you know better, you can choose better!

The Dangers of Artificial Colors

I have zero tolerance for artificial colors. I don't eat products with artificial colors or allow them in my children's diet at all. This may sound extreme—but there are so many reasons why we shouldn't be eating them, especially children. Artificial colors:

- Have been shown to disrupt the immune system. Research has found that "The molecules of synthetic colorants are small, and the immune system finds it difficult to defend the body against them. They can also bond to food or body proteins and, thus, are able to act in stealth mode to circumvent and disrupt the immune system." [25]

- May harm children's health and best be avoided according to a 2018 American Academy of Pediatrics (AAP) policy statement. [26]

- Have been banned in countries such as Norway and Austria. [27] Titanium dioxide was more recently banned in Europe due to studies linking it to genotoxicity, which is the ability to damage DNA. [28]

- Are known to cause an increase in hyperactivity in children, which requires a warning label in Europe that states "May have an adverse effect on activity and attention in children." [29]

- Can be contaminated with known carcinogens (a.k.a. an agent directly involved in causing cancer). [30]

- Have a negative impact on children's ability to learn.

- Have been linked to long-term health problems such as asthma, skin rashes, and migraines.

- Do not change the flavor of food and add absolutely no nutritional value to the foods we are eating. They are used solely for aesthetic purposes. There are safer alternatives.

Worst Drinks for Kids

The unhealthiest drinks are also the most popular among children. It saddens me greatly that most children have at least one of these in their lunch boxes every day, and then drink more of them at home too. These drinks are filled with either extreme amounts of refined sugar or artificial sweeteners made in a lab. They also contain processed preservatives and other additives. Sodas are at the top of the list, especially fruit-flavored sodas and so-called "juice" drinks that contain artificial dyes. This is not an exhaustive list, but includes specific drinks and brands commonly served to children.

- Sunkist Orange Soda
- Crush Grape Soda
- Jarritos fruit sodas
- A&W Root Beer
- Sprite
- 7UP
- Little Hug Fruit Barrels
- Hi-C

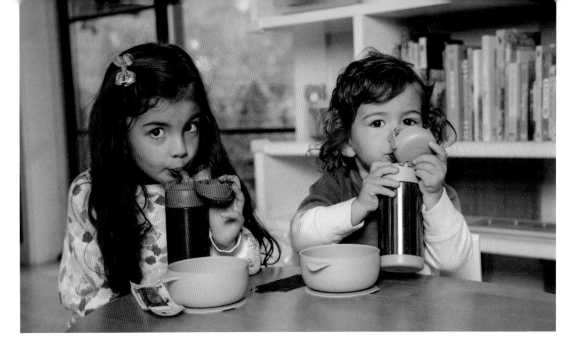

- Hawaiian Punch
- Sunkist Strawberry Lemonade
- Gatorade
- Gatorade Zero
- Powerade
- Powerade Zero
- Kool-Aid Jammers
- Kool-Aid Jammers Zero Sugar
- Kool-Aid Bursts
- Sparkling Ice
- Splash Blast Flavored Water
- Capri Sun
- Nesquik Strawberry
- Nesquik Chocolate
- Carnation Breakfast Essentials Ready-to-Drink
- Pediasure Grow & Gain Kids' Nutritional Shake

Not-Much-Better Drinks for Kids

I'd categorize these drinks as slightly better than soda, but still not great for children. This is where most "juice boxes" fall—they are loaded with juice "concentrates" and added flavors and preservatives. Most of these drinks are also not made with organic fruit, which means that they are more likely to be contaminated with pesticides.

- Snapple juice drinks
- V8 Splash juices
- Simply Light Orange Juice
- Danimals Smoothies
- Good2grow 100% juice products
- Minute Maid 100% juice products
- Minute Maid Kids+ juices
- Juicy Juice 100% juice products
- Mott's Mighty juice drinks
- Ocean Spray Growing Goodness juices

Still-Not-the-Best Drinks for Kids

The drinks in this category are much better than the majority of kid-marketed drinks, but they're not ideal. Even some of the organic products listed below are made from juice concentrates, making them high in sugar. Most of them are spiked with natural flavors, which are proprietary mixtures designed in a lab, so you don't know what you are drinking. I'm also not a fan of drinking out of cans, which is how most flavored waters are packaged. That's because the lining used in cans can disrupt hormones.

- Apple & Eve Organics 100% juice boxes
- Honest Kids organic juice boxes
- RETHINK Juice Splash boxes
- RETHINK organic flavored water boxes
- Zevia Kidz zero-calorie soda (canned)
- Creative Roots flavored coconut water
- Uncle Matt's Organic No Sugar Added Lemonade boxes
- Santa Cruz Organic juices
- R. W. Knudsen organic juices
- Clearly Canadian sparkling water
- Hint Kids infused water boxes
- Waterloo sparkling water (canned)
- Bubly sparkling water (canned)
- LaCroix sparkling water (canned)
- Spindrift flavored water (canned)

Best Drinks for Kids

I breastfed Harley until she was three and a half years old, and I still breastfeed my two-year-old, so conventional dairy and sugary drinks were easy to avoid. The drinks listed below are what I feel most comfortable drinking myself and serving my kids. Filtered water is the main drink in my house, and sometimes we make our own flavored water for my six-year-old. To do this, you start with filtered water (flat or sparkling) and squeeze in your own orange, lemon or lime slices, and/or slices of other fruits such as watermelon, cucumber, and strawberries. These homemade drinks are great to pair with coconut water or a little honey if your kids are under the weather too. Any juices listed below are organic, cold pressed, and not from concentrate. They are still high in natural sugars, so it's a good idea to mix these with water for your child. This is a money-saver too! Milk is a beverage and not a nutritional requirement. If you choose to serve your child milk, it's healthiest to choose raw organic milk if available to you.

- Filtered water
- Homemade flavored water with fresh fruit or vegetables
- Mountain Valley spring water (glass bottles)
- MALK unsweetened nondairy milks
- Harmless Harvest organic coconut water
- GT's Organic Synergy Raw Kombucha

- Evolution Fresh organic cold-pressed juices
- Uncle Matt's Organic Orange Juice
- Lakewood organic PURE juices
- Biotta organic beet juice
- Organic grass-fed whole milk
- Raw grass-fed milk
- Numi Organic Moroccan Mint Tea
- Numi or Traditional Medicinals organic chamomile tea
- Other non-caffeinated organic herbal teas

Healthier Packaged Foods for Busy Parents

While I always advocate eating mostly homemade whole foods, there are some packaged options that are a good choice and are more convenient than making everything from scratch. Instead of buying full meals that are packaged, I recommend buying some components that can make putting a meal together easy. For example, instead of buying Gerber Spaghetti Rings or SpaghettiOs, cook some lentil pasta and top it with Lucini pasta sauce and some Parmesan cheese. I like to add some diced kale to the sauce or some shredded and cooked veggies for additional nutrition. You can package it in small freezable jars to store in the freezer, so you always have your own "packaged" food ready to go.

Below you'll find my favorite brands that I often stock in my own kitchen. You'll find these in natural food grocery stores and online.

Almond Butter (or any Nut Butter)
- Artisana Raw Organic Nut Butters
- Wilderness Poets Raw Organic Nut Butters
- MaraNatha Raw Organic Nut Butters

Almond Milk (or any Nut Milk or Oat Milk)
- Malk Organic Nut Milks
- Three Trees Nut Milks

BBQ Sauce
- Mother Raw Organic BBQ Sauce
- Primal Kitchen Organic BBQ Sauce
- Kinder's Organic BBQ Sauce
- Date Lady Organic BBQ Sauce
- Bone Broth
- Bonafide Provisions Organic Bone Broth (Frozen)

Bread
- Ezekiel Organic Sprouted Bread
- Organic Bread of Heaven (mail order)
- One Degree Organic Breads
- Happy Campers Organic Breads (gluten free)
- Dave's Killer Bread

Cake Mix

- Miss Jones Organic Cake Mix
- Simple Mills Cake Mix
  (gluten free)
  Namaste Foods Organic
  Cake Mix (gluten free)

Crackers

- Mary's Gone Organic Crackers
- Edward & Sons Black Sesame
  Brown Rice Snaps

Freeze-Dried Fruit

- Natierra freeze-dried fruit

Frozen Fruit

- A variety of organic frozen
  fruit like berries and pineapple
  that you can quickly blend
  into a smoothie.

Frozen Vegetables

- A variety of organic frozen
  vegetables like peas, lima beans,
  and diced butternut squash.

Fruit Leather

- Solely Organic Fruit Jerky
- Peaceful Fruits Organic
  Fruit Strips

Granola

- One Degree Sprouted Granola
- Purely Elizabeth Granola

Guacamole

- Whole Foods Fresh Guacamole

Hot Cocoa Mix

- Nibmor

Hummus

- Hope Organic Hummus

Ice Cream

- Cosmic Bliss

Jam

- Crofter's Organic Fruit Spread
- LOOV Organic Fruit Spread
- Bionaturae Organic Fruit Spread

Ketchup

- Primal Kitchen Organic Ketchup

Mayonnaise

- Chosen Foods Avocado Oil Mayo
- Primal Kitchen Avocado Oil Mayo

Pancake/Waffle Mix

- Arrowhead Mills Organic
  Buckwheat Pancake & Waffle Mix
- Bob's Red Mill 7 Grain Organic
  Pancake & Waffle Mix
- Birch Benders Organic
  and Gluten Free

Pasta Sauce

- Lucini Organic Pasta Sauces

Peanut Butter

- MaraNatha Organic Peanut Butter
- Santa Cruz Organic Peanut Butter
- Trader Joe's Organic Peanut Butter
- Once Again Organic Peanut Butter

Pasta

- Chickapea Organic Pasta
- Jovial Organic Pasta

Popcorn

- Lesser Evil Organic Popcorn
- Trader Joe's Organic Olive Oil Popcorn

Pickles

- Grillo's Pickles

Pizza Crust

- Simple Mills Pizza Crust Mix
- Essential Baking Company Organic Pizza Crust

Pizza Sauce

- Whole Foods 365 Organic Pizza Sauce
- Simple Truth Organic Pizza Sauce
- Primal Kitchen Organic Pizza Sauce

Popsicles

- Good Pop Organic Frozen Pops

Pretzels

- Hanover Organic Ancient Grains Spelt Pretzels

Ranch Dip

- Primal Kitchen Organic Ranch Dip

Rice Cakes

- Suzie's Thin rice cakes
- Lundberg Family Farms brown rice cakes

Salad Dressing

- Mother Raw Organic Salad Dressings
- Primal Kitchen Organic Salad Dressings
- Bragg Organic Salad Dressing

Salsa

- Field Day Organic Salsas

Seasoning Mixes

- Simply Organic Seasoning Mixes
- Noble Made Organic Seasonings

Snack Bars

- Truvani The Only Bar
- Kate's Real Food Bars

Teriyaki Sauce

- Coconut Secret
- Big Tree Farms

Tortillas (Flour)

- Organic Bread of Heaven Tortillas (mail order)
- Ezekiel Organic Sprouted Grain Tortillas
- Siete Tortillas (gluten free)

Tortillas (Corn)

- Ezekiel Organic Sprouted Corn Tortillas

Veggie Burgers

- Hilary's Organic Veggie Burgers

PROCESSED FOOD SWAPS!

When we became parents we made the decision to not have any processed junk food in the house. So my children aren't growing up with the typical Capri Suns in the fridge, Cheetos in the pantry, and Lovebird Honey Cereal in the cabinets. I've figured out how to replace Fruit by the Foot and all the typical junk food that children eat with either carefully selected store-bought swaps or easy homemade recipes. Here I provide several examples of how to do this. There are not identical swaps for everything, and the alternative may not perfectly resemble the original, as we try to keep white sugars and white flours out of our diets as much as possible, and use much healthier ingredients.

Breakfast Foods

Cocoa Krispies Cereal

Alternative: One Degree Organic Sprouted Brown Rice Cacao Crisps (still contains 10 grams added coconut sugar per serving, so use very sparingly)

Eggo French Toast Sticks

Alternative: Fun with Shapes French Toast recipe on page 90

Honey Bunches of Oats Granola

Alternative #1: Purely Elizabeth Organic Granola

Alternative #2: Homemade Granola (recipe inside *Food Babe Kitchen*)

Lovebird Honey Cereal

Alternative: One Degree Organic Sprouted Oat Honey O's (still contains 3 grams added sugar, so use sparingly)

Little Bites Mini Muffins

Alternative: Pumpkin Muffins recipe on page 115

Nutri-Grain Bars

Alternative: Goji Berry Breakfast Cookies recipe on page 97

Quaker Instant Oatmeal Packets

Alternative: On-the-Go Protein Oatmeal Jars recipe on page 108

Toaster Strudels

Alternative: Copycat Toaster Strudel recipe on page 278

Unicorn Eggo Waffles

Alternative: Fast Green Waffles recipe on page 105

Snack Foods

Danimals Yogurt

Alternative: Whole grassfed organic yogurt or coconut yogurt mixed with pureed fruit

Dole Fruit Bowls & Parfait Cups

Alternative: Chia Seed Fruit Salad recipe on page 102

Doritos and Chips

Alternative #1: Cheeze It Up Brad's Crunchy Kale

Alternative #2: Crispy Ranch Chickpeas recipe on page 160

Fruit Snacks

Alternative: Dried fruit such as prunes, cherries, apricots, mangos, raisins, etc.

Fruit by the Foot

Alternative: Real Food Fruit Leather recipe on page 180

GoGurt Yogurt

Alternative: Sweet Nothings Organic Squeezable Smoothies

Goldfish and Cheez-It Crackers

Alternative #1: Simple Mills Cheddar Crackers

Alternative #2: Cheesy Crackers recipe on page 176

Hot Pockets

Alternative: Homemade "Hot Pockets" recipe on page 179

Pizza Rolls

Alternative #1: Snow-Days Grain-Free Pizza Bites

Alternative #2: Zucchini Pizza Bites recipe on page 164

Waffle Fries

Alternative: Copycat "Chick-fil-A" Waffle Fries recipe on page 244

Lunch and Dinner

Campbell's Tomato Soup

Alternative: Homemade Tomato Kale Soup recipe on page 188

Chicken Nuggets

Alternative: "Chick-fil-A" Chicken Nuggets recipe on page 210

Kraft Mac & Cheese

Alternative: Lentil pasta or whole wheat pasta with butter and shredded cheese

Lunchables

Alternative: Applegate Organic Deli Turkey cut into smaller pieces, organic cheese cut into square slices, green olives, and Jovial Organic Sourdough Einkorn Crackers or Mary's Gone Organic Real Thin Crackers

SpaghettiOs

Alternative: Lentil Pasta with Zucchini and Tomato Sauce recipe on page 150

Totino's Party Pizza

Alternative: Quick and Easy Home-Baked Pizza recipe on page 228

Drinks

Capri Sun drinks and other juice boxes

Alternative: Homemade flavored water—squeeze in fresh fruit (such as orange slices)

Gatorade

Alternative: Homemade Sports Drink recipe on page 134

Nesquik Chocolate Milk

Alternative #1: Chocolate PB Superfood Smoothie recipe on page 126

Alternative #2: Chocolate Kiki Milk

Sprite and 7UP

Alternative: Lemon-Lime Fizz recipe on page 137

Desserts

Baskin-Robbins Ice Cream

Alternative: Banana Split recipe on page 285

Chips Ahoy!

Alternative: Simple Mills or Jovial Organic Cookies

Ice Cream Cups

Alternative: Sweet Nothings Smoothie Cups

Jell-O Cups

Alternative: Key Lime Pie Parfait recipe on page 111

Keebler Cookies

Alternative: Siete Cookies

Little Debbie Oatmeal Cream Pies

Alternative: Oatmeal Cream Pie Cookies recipe on page 280

Oreos

Alternative: Homemade "Oreos" recipe on page 276

Popsicles

Alternative: Superfood Pops recipe on page 270

Snack Pack Pudding Cups

Alternative: 5-Minute Chocolate Pudding Cups recipe on page 274

Swiss Miss Hot Cocoa

Alternative: 3-Ingredient Hot Cocoa Mix recipe on page 141

RADICAL OPINION: KIDS DON'T NEED GOLDFISH CRACKERS

Almost every child in the United States eats Goldfish crackers. It is the second most popular cracker brand in the country, and American families are consuming more than 150 billion Goldfish crackers each year—which has gone up exponentially in recent years.[31] It's quite astonishing when you think about how popular these little cheese crackers are. Parents buy giant boxes of Goldfish at Costco to pack in their children's lunch boxes. Soccer moms stash them in their car to share on the field. Preschools and daycares serve them and keep Goldfish on their list of acceptable snacks for parents to pack for their children. How has Pepperidge Farm mesmerized parents and caregivers everywhere into believing that this is a good snack for their children?

The Snack That Smiles Back

Much of the allure of Goldfish crackers has to do with successful marketing campaigns that fuel the idea that these crackers are a convenient tasty snack that children love. They're available to buy in ready-to-go snack-size bags—all a parent needs to do is pop one in their backpack, and voila! However, it turns out that Pepperidge Farm had even more tricks up their sleeve. They have been slyly targeting your children for several decades. In the mid-1990s Pepperidge Farm consulted with experimental social psychologist Marianne LaFrance to help make their products more attractive to children. Their research uncovered that children are drawn to smiling faces and concluded they needed to incorporate this into their product. That is when they added a friendly smile to the Goldfish, becoming the "Snack That Smiles Back." Now we see they were right on the money! Babies and toddlers everywhere are drawn to these smiling cheddar fish, and eat them by the handful.

What's the Harm, *Really*?

Goldfish seem healthier than other snacks like Cheetos. Advertisements tells us they are baked, never fried, and made with real cheese. But let's take a look at the ingredient label.

Goldfish Cheddar Crackers: Enriched Wheat Flour (Flour, Niacin, Reduced Iron, Thiamine Mononitrate, Riboflavin, Folic Acid), Cheddar Cheese ([Cultured Milk, Salt, Enzymes], Annatto), Vegetable Oils (Canola, Sunflower And/Or Soybean), Salt, Contains 2% Or Less Of: Yeast, Sugar, Autolyzed Yeast Extract, Paprika, Spices, Celery, Onion Powder, Monocalcium Phosphate, Baking Soda.

The first and most abundant ingredient in Goldfish is "enriched wheat flour." As you remember from the Terrible 10 ingredients on page 29, this is essentially dead food. Pepperidge Farm makes a separate version of Goldfish crackers with "whole wheat flour" as the first ingredient. Whole wheat flour is more nutritious for the body in terms of nutrients because the entire wheat germ is used and not discarded like it is in processing white flour. However, it's still very processed, and manufacturers have the option to use a myriad of chemicals to extend the shelf life. The wheat germ has natural oils in it, allowing fresh milled flour to last only a few months before it goes bad. Obviously, food manufacturers do whatever they can to prevent this, even if it means making the food less nutritious.

"Baked with Real Cheese"?

The second most abundant ingredient in Goldfish crackers is conventional cheddar cheese. This means the cheese is not organic. Pepperidge Farm makes one version of Goldfish with "organic wheat flour," but none of the other ingredients are organic, including the cheese. There are currently no Goldfish on the market with organic cheese. This is an issue because non-organic cheese comes from some very controversial farming processes. Conventional cheese comes from large factory farms where the cows are raised on an unhealthy diet of GMO feed that is likely sprayed with glyphosate and other cancerous pesticides. Additionally, the cows may be administered synthetic hormones that are linked to cancer. These chemicals can end up in their milk and other dairy products such as conventional cheese. Conventional dairy cows are commonly given antibiotics to treat mastitis (udder infections). Farmers are supposed to ensure the antibiotics have left their system before producing milk, but this isn't always the case as residues have been found in conventional milk sold in stores, while none was found in the organic milk that was tested.[32] The overuse of antibiotics on farms is causing antibiotic-resistant bacteria to proliferate, and pretty soon, it may be that when you get an infection, antibiotics won't work for you.

This is a very scary problem. Organic cows are fed 100 percent organic feed and are not administered synthetic hormones. If an organic cow requires antibiotics, it is treated and removed from organic production so that its milk cannot be used in organic products. For all these reasons, I think it is very important to choose organic dairy products, and refuse to buy products like Goldfish that are made with conventional cheese.

Goldfish are cooked with three different vegetable oils: canola, sunflower, and soybean oil. All three of these oils are heavily processed and refined. In the factories where they are produced, they go through an insane amount of processing with chemical solvents, steamers, neutralizers, dewaxers, bleach, and deodorizers before they end up in our food. The solvent that is most often used to extract the oil is the neurotoxin hexane—the seeds and soybeans are literally bathed in it. Besides how extremely processed these vegetable oils are, they are also not healthy for your body. Soybean and sunflower oils specifically are extraordinarily high in omega-6 fatty acids, and while our bodies need this type of fatty acid, today people are getting way too much of it through processed foods—up to 20 times more than required. The overabundance of omega-6 fatty acids in the diet increases the risk of inflammation, cardiovascular disease, cancer, and autoimmune diseases.

The Hidden Ingredient That Makes Goldfish Irresistible

It turns out that to make that cheesy flavor everyone craves, it takes more than just cheese. Pepperidge Farm adds the little-known ingredient "autolyzed yeast extract" to Goldfish crackers. This is an additive used to make food addicting, and the reason why it is so powerful is because it is simply MSG disguised under another name. As discussed in the Terrible 10 ingredients on page 29, this is purely used to increase food cravings and irresistibility, to keep you coming back for more.

When you combine the blood sugar–spiking ingredient white flour, with cheap oils and an addictive flavoring chemical—you create the perfect food for hooking your child's brain to crave it over and over again. I personally don't want my child's taste buds to be hijacked by foods spiked with chemicals like this. I don't want to foster the habit of munching on low-quality processed foods, which can eventually lead to diseases like obesity, heart disease, diabetes, and cancer later in life.

What You Won't Find on the Label

In 2016, an FDA-registered food safety laboratory was commissioned by The Detox Project and Food Democracy Now to test popular American food products for residues of the weed killer glyphosate (Roundup).[33] They specifically found this weed killer in Goldfish. In three samples of Goldfish tested, they detected 18.40 ppb glyphosate in Goldfish Original crackers, 8.02 ppb in Goldfish Colors crackers, and 24.58 ppb in Goldfish Whole Grain crackers. While these amounts are not as large as other products tested, and we don't know if Goldfish crackers are still tainted, I don't personally feel

safe feeding my child a food known to have been contaminated with glyphosate weed killer, a chemical strongly linked to cancer. Glyphosate contamination is especially a risk whenever you buy a product that is made with non-organic wheat, since conventional wheat crops are sometimes sprayed with it before harvest, because it acts as a drying agent. That is how it ended up in products like Goldfish crackers—but you'll never see this on the label.

Better Options

If I resist the Big Food industry in only one way it would be this: I refuse to buy junk food that has no nutritional value and is designed to be addictive. And, therefore, I refuse to feed my children Goldfish crackers. Our kids will be just fine without Goldfish. Let me prove it to you. I put together a list of over 100 packaged snacks that are a zillion times better than Goldfish. You'll find it at FoodBabe.com/resources. It's time to stop encouraging children everywhere to get hooked on nutrition-less dead food! Big Food has done enough damage to our health and the future health of our children. Let's break their control together.

Now that we learned how to spot ridiculous food labels on children's food and which Terrible 10 ingredients to avoid when shopping for food, it's time to move on to how to bring it all together. In the next chapter, we'll talk about what to do at home to help foster a love for real food in your children. This is where we get into the real nitty-gritty of how to incorporate real food and healthy habits into your daily life.

Are Veggie Straws Healthier Than Chips?

I hate to break the news if you love Veggie Straws, but we need to discuss this wildly popular snack that many children (and adults) eat by the bagful. I know that having *veggie* in the name makes them sound good for you, but please look at the ingredients:

Sensible Portions Veggie Straws: Potato Starch, Potato Flour, Expeller Pressed Canola Oil And/Or Safflower Oil and/or Sunflower Oil, Spinach Powder, Tomato Paste, Salt, Cane Sugar, Corn Starch, Potassium Chloride, Turmeric (Color), Beetroot Powder (Color), Sea Salt.

As you see, Veggie Straws are mostly made from conventional potatoes and fried in vegetable oils, just like potato chips are. Let's compare them to the ingredients in Ruffles.

Ruffles Potato Chips: Potatoes, Vegetable Oil (Canola, Corn, Soybean, and/or Sunflower Oil), And Salt.

The main ingredients are very similar aren't they? The "spinach powder" and "tomato paste" in Veggie Straws primarily add color to the straws, but not much nutrition. The label says "beetroot powder" and "turmeric" are solely added for color. This doesn't make the product any more of a "veggie"—just prettier.

Most people are buying non-organic Veggie Straws, but there is an organic version found at some grocery stores. Although it's organic, it is not much better, made with processed corn and potato flour fried in unhealthy refined oils that are high in omega-6 fatty acids (which can lead to inflammation).

A great alternative to Veggie Straws are . . . real vegetables. Granted, raw vegetable strips are very different in taste and texture than chips. But dehydrated veggies can be a bridge between the two.

Want even more healthy snack ideas? Go to FoodBabe.com/resources for a list of over 100 store-bought snacks I love that are made without refined flours or processed sugars.

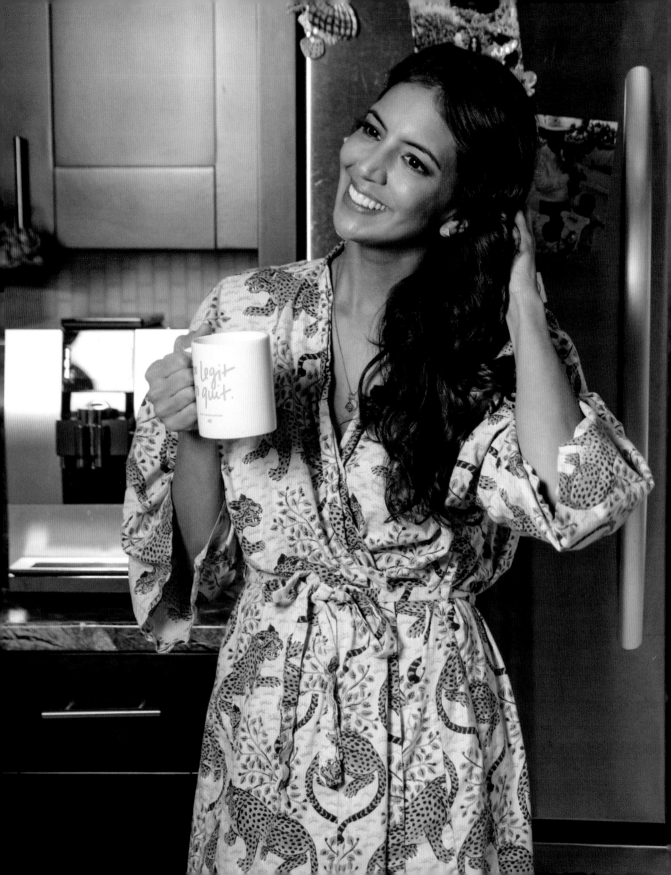

chapter 3

WHAT TO DO AT HOME

MAKING REAL FOOD FUN

When Harley was three, I was working on a campaign about Kellogg's Unicorn Waffles, which are made with artificial colors, artificial flavors, and other very processed ingredients. Harley came into my office, sat on my lap, and saw the graphic I was creating. Her face lit up when she saw that colorful purple box with a rainbow unicorn and pink waffles on it, and she exclaimed, "Mom, *mmm* those waffles look good!" And, of course they did. Those colorful boxes are very enticing to any young child; that's exactly what Kellogg's is banking on and how they are able to sell boxes by the truckload. I used this as a learning opportunity and talked to her about how they make waffles this pretty pink color by putting fake colors in them that aren't actually real food, and that actually those fake colors are not good for our bodies and can make us sick. You'd be amazed at how quickly young children pick up on this and understand, and now, whenever Harley sees brightly colored food she knows to ask if it is artificially colored.

This also got me thinking about ways that I could make real food fun for her to eat. If we're competing with Kellogg's—we've got to have a few tricks up our sleeve, right? So I bought these Halloween toothpicks with little pumpkin faces and Frankenstein on them, and I put one of these in her homemade pancakes or French toast. This is one way to make her meals more fun, without artificially dyed sprinkles and other things with nasty ingredients. I've also shown her how we can make food more fun and colorful by using real food, which is what you'll find in the Fast Green Waffles recipe on page 105. It incorporates spinach in the waffles to turn them green, but you'd never guess!

Here are a few more ideas:

- String berries and melons on skewers in a fun pattern. Children love to pull them off and eat kebabs.

- Let your children help in the kitchen. Kids love to get involved in what you're doing! See my best tips for this on pages 57–58.

- Use a cookie cutter to cut foods into fun shapes. This works well with waffles, pancakes, cheese, melons, cucumber, and sandwiches.

- Set up a salad bar. Wash and prepare all of the makings for a salad in separate containers and let your child create their own salad bowl. You can do something similar for other dishes too, such as wraps, smoothies, tacos, pizza, etc.

- Children love to dip! Soups, hummus, dressings, and nut butters all make great dips for veggies, crackers, and breads. You'll find my favorite dip recipes in Kid Snacks on page 159.

- Use real food to add color to foods. You can buy powders made out of 100 percent freeze-dried produce to add color to waffles, cakes, cookies, pancakes, and other dishes. This way you can avoid artificial dyes and boost nutrition too! For example, you can use freeze-dried dragon fruit powder or strawberry powder to color your own pink "Unicorn Waffles."

- Create a theme night. For instance, you can have a "princess night" where you prepare food for princesses and decorate the table with a few princess decorations. Put on some of their favorite princess music and have fun with it. You can do this for any character or hobby that your child is into.

- Take your children on foodie field trips. Let them explore your local pumpkin patches and pick from apple trees in the fall, pick berries at a u-pick farm in the summer, and shop at the farmer's market to pick out their favorite smoothie ingredients.

- Use food to create a fun smiling face. For instance, if you are serving your child a pancake, you can decorate it with banana slices for the eyes and nose and strawberry slices for the smile. This helps motivate a child to try eating more fruit. This idea works well with homemade mini-pizzas, English muffins, rice cakes, and waffles. You can make flowers, spirals, and other fun designs with the toppings.

IS YOUR CHILD REALLY "PICKY"?

Many children are labeled as "picky" eaters when they are very young. The first time a baby turns up their nose at a jar of Gerber pureed peas, the parents decide that they hate peas and never offer them peas again. Even when this baby becomes a toddler, the parents remember that they "hate peas" and don't ever put them on their plate. When their child later makes a funny face after tasting bitter broccoli, the parents decide their child also hates broccoli and add it to the growing list of foods they won't eat. This greatly influences future food choices, and next thing you know you've decided that your child hates all vegetables. They will likely be convinced of this as well. Don't be so quick to assume.

It's normal for children to fear new foods when they are little. Even if they've tried something many times, they may suddenly stop wanting to eat it for a while, but this doesn't mean they hate the food. Children are born with an innate dislike for bitter flavors, which are found in many vegetables such as broccoli, kale, and arugula. As Bettina Elias Siegel writes in her book, *Kid Food*, this is likely because bitterness is a signal in the wild that a plant might be poisonous, so this is a protective mechanism.[1] Thankfully, most children outgrow this.

The first solid food that most babies are given is rice cereal. I consider this some of the worst advice. That's because it is bland and doesn't give babies interesting flavors to explore from the get-go. It's best to start out early with flavorful vegetables, moving on to fruits, and then proteins. I go into great detail about how I did this with my own children on pages 4–5. During their first few bites of solid food (around four to seven months old) is when babies are most receptive to new flavors, so you don't want to miss this opportunity.

When your child spits food out or throws it across the room, it may look like they hate it, but don't give up. It's been shown that children may need multiple exposures to new foods before they will eat them. Sometimes as many as 10 or even 15 times! If you fall back on offering processed favorites all the time, like mac n' cheese and chicken nuggets filled with MSG and natural flavors, you are reinforcing a love for processed food and making it less likely that your child will want to eat real food and vegetables in the future. Likewise, it can backfire if you are putting too much pressure on your child by forcing them to eat their vegetables before they can have something they already enjoy eating. Balance is always important.

Ultimately, you decide what food your children will be served at mealtimes. It's up to your child whether or not they will actually eat it. This allows your child to feel in control of their diet, although you are the one providing the options. Let them choose between two vegetables, for instance— green beans or carrots—along with other items in the meal that they enjoy eating. If they choose not to eat either of the vegetables, don't worry about it and try again at another meal. Keep trying. Remember 10 to 15 exposures may be the magic number that you need! Be careful not to label your child as picky, because they just might grow up to meet your expectations.

Encouraging Your Child to Try New Foods

Get your kids involved in choosing meals and ingredients. Ask them to help you make a weekly meal plan, picking out their favorite recipes from the choices you give them. You can bring them to the store with you to buy the ingredients and pick out the best and brightest produce for the dinner you're making. Give them a job in the kitchen too; helping you prepare and cook dinner really gets them invested in the process and more excited to eat what you have all created.

Read fun books about healthy food together. It's more fun to read a story about a character who eats spinach and gets stronger than it is to simply tell your child to eat more spinach. From a very early age you can start talking to your child about the health benefits of certain foods in terms that they will understand, and reading fun books makes it very memorable for young children.

Explain why healthy foods are good for them. This gives them incentive to want to try healthy food. Don't just simply say, "Blueberries are healthy." It's better to give them a little fact to chew on, even if they are really young, such as, "Blueberries are great for your heart" or "Carrots help you see clearly" or "Oranges help keep you from getting sick." As they get older, expand on this a bit and give them more reasons, like,

"Blueberries have a lot of antioxidants in them that are like little warriors in your body, which helps keep your heart healthy."

Make healthy food fun! Use fun dips and other strategies to make healthy food look more interesting and fun to eat. You won't need to do this forever as your kids will grow out of it soon enough. Check out my tips on pages 49–50.

Don't pressure them. When children are pressured, their response is typically to push back and refuse whatever you are pushing them to do. This can backfire and encourage bad habits. Allow your child to feel safe about choosing what they want to eat. Remember that you are responsible for providing healthy food for your child, but they can decide whether or not they will eat it. Instead of playing games, forcing them to try a bite, or nagging them to eat their cauliflower, simply serve them the cauliflower with the rest of their meal. If they don't eat it, tell them that is okay (and try it again later). Constantly providing healthy options is key here.

Try and try again. The first time your child is exposed to a new food, they are exploring it. They might give it a lick. They might take a bite and spit it out. They might not even taste it at all, and throw it across the room in disgust. This may feel disheartening, but remember this is a totally normal learning experience for children. I can't reiterate it enough that you simply don't want to give up. Continue offering the food multiple times, without pressure, and it is very likely that they will eventually give it a try and may even love it.

Add vegetables to their favorite items. If your child loves nut butter, spread it on celery sticks. If your child loves hummus with crackers, add a few veggie sticks to the plate or blend veggies into their hummus. If they love quesadillas or pizzas, add vegetables to them. Think about other ways you can add vegetables to their favorite foods.

Keep servings small. Start out with small servings and add more to their plates only when they ask for more. Small portions are less overwhelming visually and that alone can encourage your children to take a bite of something new. This approach also helps you waste less food!

Limit snack time. If your child isn't eating healthy foods at lunch and dinner, it could be because they are eating snacks too close to mealtimes. Children will be more open to eating a variety of food when they are hungry. So, don't offer them snacks all the time. Keep the kitchen closed between meals and offer them snacks only if it's been a couple hours since their last meal and another couple hours before their next meal. In other words, there should be a couple hours after a snack before you serve a meal. This also goes for bedtime snacks. If your child knows they'll be getting a snack before bed, they may skip out on their dinner and hold out for a bedtime snack. As I mentioned earlier, we had to add a safety lock to our pantry door because our little one thought the pantry

was an all-day, all-you-can-eat buffet! Simply adding the lock helped set the boundary that snacks are only appropriate at snack time and need approval from a parent.

Be positive. If you're stressed out about establishing healthy eating habits or scared that your child won't like a new vegetable, they will pick up on your stress and fear, and that alone could make them resistant. Simply present a new food to them in a positive and open way, and give them the choice of whether or not they will eat it, taste it, or refuse it altogether.

Don't blame yourself. There are so many factors involved. Every child is unique and will develop at their own rate. Some children will take longer than others to enjoy certain foods, and some may never like a certain food. It's not your fault and doesn't make you a bad parent! Children will grow and thrive even if their diet is not perfect, so don't put so much pressure on yourself.

5 WAYS TO HELP YOUR CHILD LOVE GREEN DRINKS

I don't remember ever eating vegetables when I was little. (Sorry, Mom! I know you tried!) As a result, I went years without some of the best nutrients life has to offer. My old eating habits created havoc in my body. In my teen years and into my 20s I had stomach issues, eczema, and asthma, and my allergies were atrocious—I was constantly in and out of doctors' offices looking for a solution.

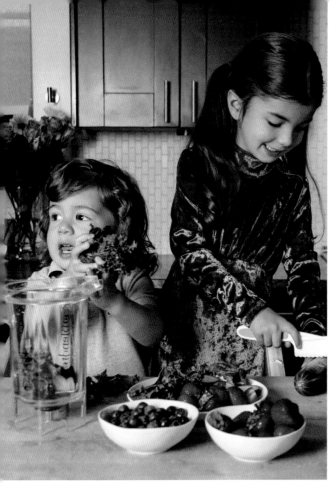

As soon as I started to investigate my food habits, I replaced all the chemical-laden processed and fast food that I had been eating with whole and organic foods, which included lots of vegetables. My health did a 180 from when I was younger! I went from being a kid always going to the doctor to enjoying a life without prescription drugs and feeling more energy than I did when I was younger. Every time I look in the mirror, it's a huge reminder of how far I've come—and there's no going back.

I began the habit of drinking a green drink every single day after I started learning about the power of green vegetables and how they can protect us from disease.

By green drink, I mean a smoothie or a juice made mostly from kale, romaine lettuce, spinach, and other leafy veggies. I can only imagine all the pain I would have eliminated if I had supplied my growing body with the nutrients it needed from green vegetables during my childhood. One of my goals is to help you avoid all this pain and foster a love for vegetables in your children. Drinking green drinks is one of the easiest habits to implement—even if your child is picky. If your child sticks their nose up at a plate of kale, they might think differently when they try it blended into a fun "Superhero Juice" with their favorite fruit. You'll find a lot of smoothie recipes in this cookbook because smoothies are the ultimate fast food. When you are a busy parent (and who isn't?) it takes no time at all to whip up a nutrient-dense smoothie for your family. Every parent needs an arsenal of smoothie recipes in their life.

To help you get started, here are six tips to encourage your children to love green drinks and convince them that greens do a body good!

1. Involve them every step of the way.

Take your child to the grocery store or farmer's market so they can help pick out the ingredients. Let them hold and smell the produce that they'd like to use in a smoothie. If you have a garden, ask them to help you plant seeds and water the greens and veggies that you are growing. Tell them that you'll be using these to make some yummy drinks. Older kids will like helping you pick out the recipes. When you make a juice or smoothie, they can help wash the ingredients and place the prepared veggies into a bowl or unplugged blender.

2. Tell them how cool it is to drink green juice.

Share with them why drinking a green drink is good for them. Explain the energy-boosting benefits that they could get from drinking green juice. Liken these benefits to their favorite superhero, cartoon character, or sports star. If you have a friend or relative that they look up to, ask them to also tell your child how cool drinking green juice is, because sometimes hearing it from someone they look up to is all a kid needs to try something new (this happened with my nephews). Tell older kids about the benefits, such as clearer skin, stronger muscles, a natural glow, and longer nails. Every time you make a drink, ask them to give it a funny name like "Green Man Super Juice" to keep it fun and exciting. For young kids, you can make a game out of it and after they drink their juice or smoothie, dress them up like a superhero to play around the house with their newfound "superpowers" from drinking superfoods! As you know, processed food companies love to add cartoon characters and sports stars to their packaging to attract children, and it works! We've got to fight fire with fire, so to speak, to make homemade food as enticing as a colorful box of Baby Shark cereal.

3. Let them pick up a fun cup and straw at the store.

Tell them that this is their special cup or straw that they'll only use to drink green juices and smoothies. Stick to it, and only let them use this cup or straw when you make your green drinks. Pretty soon they might be begging you to make a juice, just so they get to drink out of their favorite utensil.

4. Lead by example and don't sweat it.

Don't make a big deal out of drinking green drinks and keep it a positive experience. Adding too much pressure might make some kids feel leery. So, if they refuse to drink it, just say "oh well" and keep trying every day until they finally do. Remember that some kids need to be exposed to new foods 10 times before they will try it. Lead by example and drink the same green drink with them. Show them how much you love drinking yours. Some children will feel more comfortable just watching you drink it at first, and will take a sip of yours before committing to drinking their own cup. Even after they've been drinking green drinks for a while, there may be some days that they will refuse to drink it. Don't sweat it. Change up the recipes so that it's not the same every time, and just keep offering green drinks to them regularly.

5. Ease into it and sweeten it up.

While I don't normally recommend using too much fruit in a juice or smoothie, a sweeter drink can help to ease your child into it. At first use two or three servings of fruit or sweet veggies (carrot, beet). Bananas and berries are great for hiding bitter flavors, and cucumbers and celery have mild flavors that blend well into any juice or smoothie. Blend the drink well and consider diluting it with a bit of filtered water so the flavor isn't as strong and it's easier to drink. Gradually change the ratio, adding more greens and less fruit, until you eventually get it down to no more than one or two pieces of fruit in the juice or smoothie. Of course, this also depends on your child. If they are especially young or haven't been exposed to a lot of sugar, they may not have developed a taste for sweets, in which case I'd recommend starting without fruit to see how that goes.

Did you know all the smoothie recipes in this cookbook are family tested and approved? My children love every single one, or else they wouldn't have made their way into this book. If your children love peaches, start out with the Peachy Green Smoothie on page 129. If they love chocolate, try the Chocolate PB Superfood Smoothie on page 126. If they're more into

bananas, try the Banana Bread Smoothie on page 130. These recipes will help you get started and will help make living in this busy, overprocessed world a piece of cake!

TEACHING YOUR CHILDREN IN THE KITCHEN

I started talking to Harley about her food when she could crawl. When she first started walking, I noticed that she was at eye level with all the candy bars under the counter in the checkout lane, and, of course, she'd reach out to grab the shiny packages of Twix and Skittles. I'd tell her that this is junk food and not real food, hoping that this would begin to embed in her growing mind. This approach is backed by science too, as it's been shown that children are most receptive to learning about the world around them

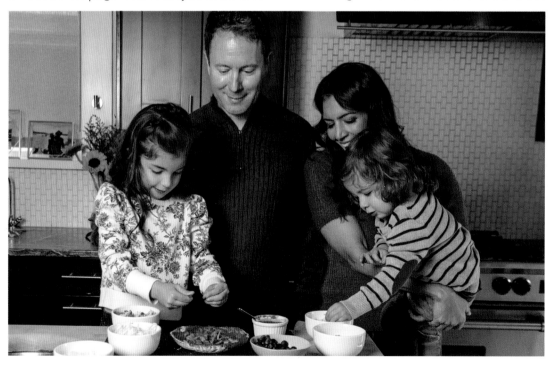

between the ages of two and seven. This is a critical period of brain development, during which they learn faster than any other time in their life.[2] You have this amazing window of time to shape their beliefs about food, so take advantage of it.

Even if your children don't seem to appreciate what you're teaching them about food now, they probably will when they're older. I recently ran into a woman I know at Berrybrook Farm (this is a natural food store in my town that I love to support, which also sells Truvani products). She told me a little trick she used with her daughters to teach them about their food. They were not allowed to pick out a product to buy at the grocery store unless they could read all of the ingredients and knew what the ingredients were. When they were little, they found this very frustrating. Can you imagine a nine-year-old trying to read the ingredients on Little Debbie Honey Buns and knowing what all those processed ingredients are? Ha! What a great lesson, right? Now her daughters are really grateful that they know what's in their food and where it comes from.

One of the best tools I bought for my kitchen when my daughter was a toddler was a Learning Tower. This is a partially enclosed wood stool that allows her to safely stand at counter height in the kitchen with us. So whenever I'm chopping up vegetables for dinner or prepping a meal, she is right there with me. Now, my son, Finley, is old enough for the Learning Tower and loves it just as much as she did. This helps our children feel like they aren't missing out on the action and I can easily give them safe activities to help

in the kitchen. This also opens up a ton of opportunities to talk about the ingredients that we're using to cook with. I tell them what different fruits and vegetables are and why they are good for you. I explain what I'm doing and how I'm cooking something, so they start to learn how to use these ingredients to make meals.

Depending on their age, your child can mix the batter, wash the vegetables, and add smoothie ingredients to a blender. There are many ways they can help, learn, and have fun in the kitchen at the same time! This will make the kitchen a comfortable place for your child where they can learn to cook when they're older. Below are a few other ways you can get them involved.

- Read recipes out loud together while you are cooking, especially in cookbooks with pictures like this one. Show them how you follow the recipe, measure out the ingredients, preheat the oven, and put it all together to make the finished product that looks like what's in the book.

- When they're old enough, they can measure out the ingredients and add them to the bowl or pot. This is a great opportunity for them to learn how measuring utensils work, and it's fun for them too.

- Younger children can wash vegetables and squeeze lemons, while older ones can learn to peel and chop up vegetables.

Get your child some child-safe knives that will allow them to learn motor skills for cutting when they're ready for it.

- If your toddler is too little to help out with a recipe, you can keep them busy by giving them some safe ingredients to play with, such as a sprig of herbs or a ball of dough. Let them play while they watch and listen to you cook in the kitchen.

- When your child is around seven years old, they might find it fun to put together some

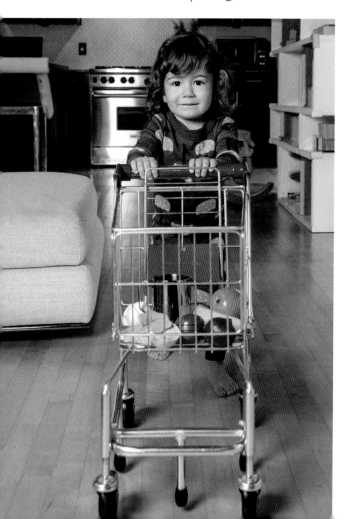

easy recipes on their own. Start with cold recipes that don't require an oven or stove, such as wraps and sandwiches.

- After they are around 10 years old, they might be ready to learn to use the stove and oven with your assistance. For instance, your child could prepare blueberry pancakes and you can show them how to safely pour the batter onto the hot griddle and flip!

- Children love to be creative, so use this to your advantage and ask them to help you decorate cookies and cakes. You can even take ordinary dishes and allow them to arrange the food on a plate in a fun way.

- Have them help set the table. Younger children can set out the napkins and older children can set the plates, glasses, and silverware.

- Ask them to help you clean up after a meal too. Show older kids how to unload and load the dishwasher or wash the pots, while younger children can wipe the table or clean up messes. Let them help scoop the leftovers into containers to store in the fridge or freezer.

Safety Tips to Remember

- Teach your child that clean hands are important. Always have them wash up before you get started in the kitchen.

- Tell them to always ask before tasting something. You don't want them licking raw chicken or eating other foods that aren't safe for them.

- Teach your child to always ask permission before cooking, especially when it comes to using the stovetop, oven, and blender or cutting up produce.

- Keep pot handles turned toward the back of the stove so their little hands don't reach up and grab them.

Above all else, keep this a positive experience for your child. It's best to involve them when you don't feel rushed so that you don't get the urge to take over when they seem to be too slow or not doing something the way you're used to doing it. Save cooking time with your child for lazy Sunday afternoons and other calmer times.

Kitchen Essentials for Children

Here are some of the kitchen tools and supplies I love. I even bring some of these items when we travel! If you don't see these in your local stores, you can find them online.

1. **Kids Learning Tower by Little Partners.** This is my favorite item in the kitchen for my kids. It allows them to stand at counter-height with me while I'm preparing food. They do all kinds of activities on the counter and it keeps them happy and busy.

2. **Stokke Tripp Trapp High Chair.**

3. **Stainless Steel Cups with Silicone Lids.** These are great because stainless steel doesn't contain endocrine-disrupting chemicals like plastic cups do.

4. **Thermos Stainless Steel Water Bottles.**

5. **Corelle Livingware Divided Dish Plates.** These are break- and chip-resistant plates—although I somehow broke one into a million pieces, so be careful!

6. **Silicone Baby Bibs.**

7. **Reusable Silicone Baking Cups.** I like to buy the normal "cupcake" size for serving snacks. The mini ones are great for baking muffins.

8. **Stainless Steel 1-Cup Bowls.**

9. **Child-Safe Cutting Knives.**

10. **Small Tempered-Glass Cups.** The ones I use are break-resistant, but you need to be careful. Glass doesn't contain potentially harmful chemicals like plastic cups do. These glasses teach children to hold and drink from a regular glass.

11. **Small Tempered-Glass Pitcher.** When they're ready, my children began pouring themselves water with this pitcher.

My Favorite Lunch Supplies for Children

- Wean Green glass containers
- LunchBots stainless steel containers
- Bentgo lunch box
- Thermos stainless steel containers

HOW TO HAVE PEACEFUL MEALS WITH YOUR FAMILY

When I was growing up, my mom never sat down to eat with us. She was always running back and forth between the kitchen and the table, keeping everything hot and fresh. She had a lot of interruptions and wasn't able to eat in peace. Now that I'm a mom, I totally get it. It's easy to be distracted with everything going on in the kitchen and making sure everyone has what they need. Sometimes it feels impossible to sit down together for a meal, but I've read so much about the incredible benefits that children get when you do this that I've made it a priority. I basically do whatever I can to make sure that we eat together regularly. It might seem old-fashioned, but our family eats dinner together every night at 5 P.M. We sit down at the table, focusing on our food while having a good conversation. We never have the TV on or our cell phones out. This is our time—undistracted and connecting with each other. I can't tell you how much I look forward to this each day.

That's not to say it's always easy to make this happen. I developed a routine and found strategies that help my family do this, and I'm going to share with you how we make this work. I compiled all of my best advice for you, but before I get into that let me point out some reasons why sitting down together to eat is so important. For starters, children who regularly sit down to eat meals with their family tend to eat fewer processed foods and more fruits and vegetables. Isn't it incredible that simply eating together can increase your child's intake of healthy food? That alone is amazing, but there are many more benefits. The conversations you are having at the dinner table are helping to improve your child's communication skills and vocabulary. It's even been shown that children get better grades in school when they regularly enjoy meals with their family. Other research finds benefits ranging from healthier body weights and higher self-esteem to stronger family relationships. The benefits apply to older children too! You may not think that teens would be interested in dining with their parents on the regular, but 80 percent of them say that family dinner is a highlight for them and that they like to use this time to talk to their parents.[3] Are you blown away yet?

If all this gives you the motivation to do what you can to regularly eat together, here are some strategies to get you there and make it fun for everyone.

- **Start with one or two meals a week.** Your meal together doesn't need to be dinner. Perhaps it's more feasible for your family to eat breakfast or lunch together. While you'll gain the most benefits if you dine together at least five times a week, it's easier to start with a smaller goal and work your way up. You have 21 different opportunities to do this each week: seven breakfasts, seven lunches, seven dinners. Pick a couple times that work for you and take it from there.

- **Anticipate what you'll need before you all sit down to eat**. This way you won't be constantly getting up to grab something. For instance, go ahead and grate the Parmesan early, put all the toppings and condiments on the table, anticipate extra silverware and napkins you might need, and cut up the fruit or dessert so it's all ready. I have a small water pitcher on the table with extra water in case my kids need more. My daughter loves using it to serve herself. Serve your dishes family style with everything on the table, so it's easy to access. Of course, keep the dishes out of reach of a toddler who might like to throw food!

- **Serve food in courses.** Instead of putting every item on your plate at once, serve your food in courses. Start with the

vegetables first, especially when your kids are small; you want to feed them what their bodies need first. Then move on to more fun dishes like the main course, breads, cheese, and proteins. Save the sweet stuff, the fruit and smoothies, for later or for dessert. When my littlest realized he would get other things he preferred after the first course, he started refusing his first course and holding out until we brought out the second course. When he pushed his plate away from him, I gently told him this is what we are having for dinner, and we all continued eating our first course. After only five minutes of watching us eat our food, he pushed his plate back to himself and started eating along with us, so we were all eating the same thing. He now knows the boundary!

- **Take your time.** Our family usually takes an entire hour to eat dinner. We don't rush it. Besides giving us a lot of time to enjoy one another's company, this gives our bodies time to healthfully process the food we're eating. Taking your time to eat also has been shown to increase fruit and vegetable consumption. Researchers studied children while they ate lunch at school and found that they ate significantly more fruit and vegetables if they were given 20 minutes to eat instead of the normal 10 minutes.[4] That's probably because children will eat their favorite foods first, which might not be the vegetables if they are rushed. If you serve your food in courses like I mentioned above, this can prolong dinner—which means you might have enough time to enjoy your meal too!

- **Put it on the calendar.** Schedule a set mealtime, write it down, share it with everyone, and try not to let events and activities interfere with this time. If necessary, it's okay to have your meal together away from home as well. For instance, you can have a picnic outdoors together before a game or practice.

- **Don't provide entertainment.** At my house we don't keep toys on the table when we're eating. Not only are children's toys probably teeming with germs, they are very distracting. Sometimes I will use a toy to get my littles to the table or they can play with them while they are waiting for dinner to be ready, but I take them off the table as the food is served. Set a rule that you will turn off the TV, iPads, laptops, and phones when you sit down for a meal. This includes banishing reading materials such as magazines—and no shuffling through your mail either. This leads to distracted, mindless eating and basically undermines all the benefits that you should be getting by eating together. Use this time to sit down with your family and connect while enjoying your food.

- **Set the mood.** While we don't allow screens, we will put on some music that our children like to listen to. This helps to keep them seated, without creating a distraction. You can also add some fun to your table with colorful place mats, fresh flowers, or other decorations.

- **Engage in positive conversation.** Keep the tone of the conversation during family meals encouraging, and don't use this time for discipline. Ask your children what good things happened during the day and share your own fun experiences. This will help your child feel heard, loved, and looking forward to this time together.

- **Invite your child to participate.** Before you sit down to eat, ask them to help set the table. Older children may be able to put the cooked dishes and other items you'll need during your meal on the table. During the meal, older children can pour drinks and help with adding servings to plates. After you're done eating, ask them to wipe up their messes and help pick up the table. They can help with those dishes too!

In the next chapter, we'll delve into how to navigate the world we live in with your child, despite it being full of processed food temptations like M&M's, Pepsi, and Doritos. I'll show you how we handle birthday parties, the food in school, holiday candy, eating in restaurants, and what we do when we travel and go to events. You obviously can't be with your child all the time and everywhere they go, so it's very important to also teach them strategies to use when faced with food decisions and challenges as they venture out on their own.

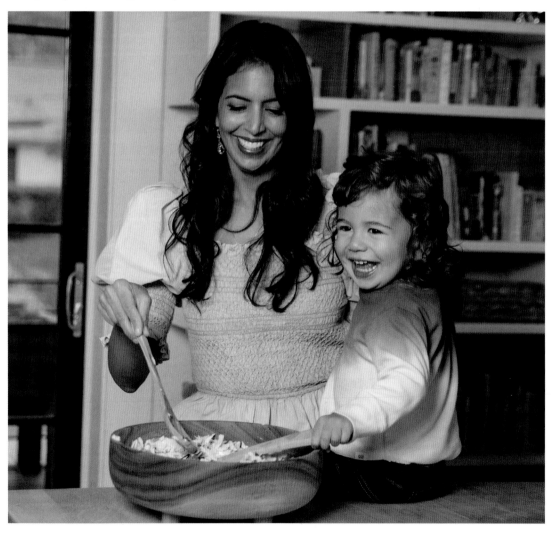

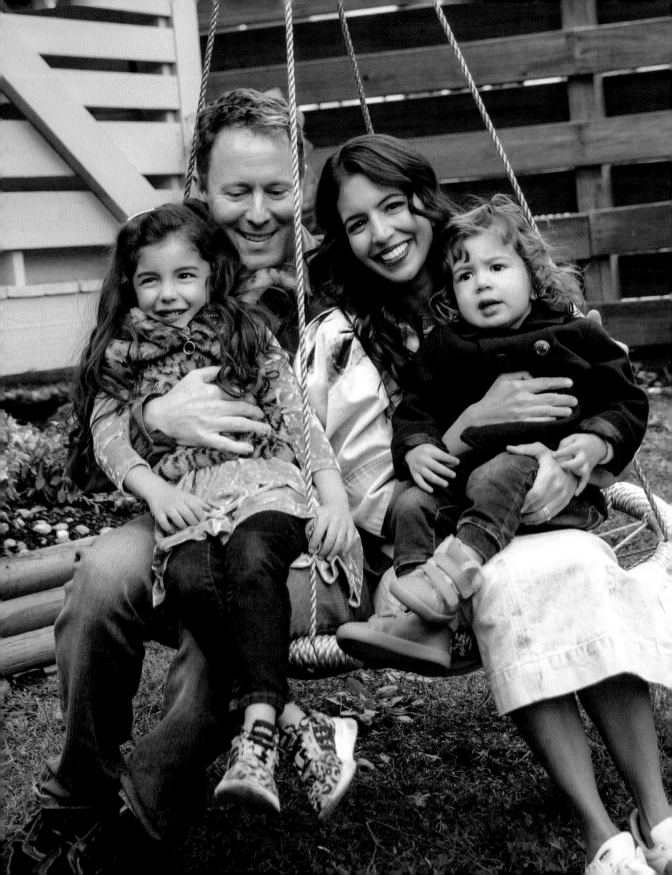

chapter 4

NAVIGATING THE OVERPROCESSED WORLD WE LIVE IN

I know you're probably wondering how you're going to apply all you've learned out in the real world. It's not easy, but I know you can do it! In this chapter I'll help you navigate the food in schools, restaurants, events, birthday parties, holidays, and while you're traveling.

SCHOOLS

I can't tell you how many moms and dads have shared with me their disgust about the food being served to their children at school. They beg me to do something to help. They ask me to start a petition or a letter-writing campaign. I could write an entire book on this subject (and someday I might) but let me get to the point. I'm right there with you. If I could wave a magic

wand and improve the food that schools are serving, I would. Unfortunately, I am not in the position to wipe the slate clean. This is a massive issue and an uphill battle that will require a united movement to make sweeping changes. That's not to say that there isn't anything we can do. Keep reading and I'll tell you how to take control of this situation for your family, and possibly help other children in the process.

If this all comes as a surprise to you, here are some hard facts about what is being served in school cafeterias across the country. You'll find a lot of refined sugar and refined oils made from genetically modified (GMO) crops in the majority of lunches. Even worse, some schools are serving up products laced with artificial colors, which are specifically linked to an increase in hyperactivity in children. This is especially alarming as this may affect their ability to pay attention and learn in class. Some lunches are laced with monosodium glutamate (MSG) or "yeast extract" (its hidden counterpart), which can fuel an addiction to processed food and overeating. Schools are actually fostering a desire for processed food in your children when they serve popular brands like Froot Loops, which are full of artificial colors; "Reduced Fat" Doritos, with even more artificial colors; Cheez-Its, which is made with a preservative (TBHQ) that is banned in some countries; and Little Bites Muffins, which are packed with controversial preservatives and emulsifiers. Children may start eating these in school and then end up begging their parents to buy these products at the grocery store. To see for yourself what's being served, the following are the ingredients in some items found in the lunchrooms at an elementary school district in Central Florida:[1]

Whole Grain Hamburger Bun: Whole White Wheat Flour, Water, Enriched Flour (Wheat Flour, Malted Barley Flour, Niacin, Iron, Thiamine Mononitrate, Riboflavin, Folic Acid), Sugar, Yeast, Wheat Gluten, Soybean Oil. Contains 2% Or Less Of The Following: Salt, Calcium Sulfate, Calcium Propionate (Preservative), Sodium Stearoyl Lactylate, Wheat Starch, Ascorbic Acid, Enzymes. (Includes GMO Ingredients Label.)

Beef Burger: Ground Beef (Not More Than 20% Fat), Salt, Caramel Color.

American Cheese: Cultured Skim Milk and Milk, Water, Sodium Citrate, Salt, Potassium Citrate, Annatto and Paprika (color), Cream, Enzymes, Sorbic Acid (preservative), Sunflower Lecithin (anti-sticking agent).

Ketchup: Tomato Concentrate Made From Red Ripe Tomatoes, Distilled Vinegar, High-Fructose Corn Syrup, Corn Syrup, Salt, Spice, Onion Powder, Natural Flavoring.

Reduced Fat Cool Ranch Doritos: Whole Corn, Corn, Vegetable Oil (Corn, Canola, And/Or Sunflower Oil), Corn Bran, Salt, Corn Starch, Tomato Powder, Lactose, Whey, Skim Milk, Onion Powder, Sugar, Garlic Powder, Monosodium Glutamate, Maltodextrin (Made from Corn), Cheddar Cheese (Milk, Cheese Cultures, Salt, Enzymes), Dextrose, Malic Acid, Corn Syrup Solids, Buttermilk, Natural and Artificial Flavors, Sodium acetate, Artificial Color (Red 40, Blue 1, Yellow 5), Spice, Citric Acid, Disodium Inosinate, and Disodium Guanylate.

Fat-Free Chocolate Milk: Nonfat milk, Liquid Sugar (Sugar, Water), Contains Less than 1% of: Cocoa (Processed with Alkali), Cocoa, Cornstarch, Salt, Carrageenan, Natural Flavor, Vitamin A Palmitate, Vitamin D3.

This is why parents must do whatever we can to pack lunches (and snacks and breakfast, if needed). This is the best way to take control and choose the ingredients and products that you're comfortable with. Of course you can't be with your children every second of the day, and there will still be times when they are exposed to processed foods at school, but having a packed lunch to start with will give them a good foundation. This book is loaded with lunch box tips and recipes to help you along the way.

Improving school food isn't easy, but it is possible. If you read the introduction to this book, you'll know that I was able to get my daughter's school to stop ordering from Domino's (which uses processed ingredients like TBHQ and sodium propionate) and switch to a much healthier organic pizza place. Go back and read this story if you haven't yet, as this will show you that change in schools is possible and that you can make a difference too. Think outside the box when it comes to food being served in your child's school. Are there any small changes you can make? Are there any specific products that you can get swapped out for a healthier alternative? Anything with artificial colors is a great place to start! You can do what I did. Come armed with research and ask directly for what you want. Get other parents involved if you need to. When you work together, you can make a difference even faster. Remember that any changes you spur will not only help your child, but other children at their school too—especially those who rely on cafeteria food for all their lunches and snacks.

RESTAURANTS

When I was child I loved eating in restaurants. Although we'd sometimes eat somewhere fancy, we mostly ate fast food. Burger King was my favorite. I had many birthday parties there and got so excited when my dad bought me their croissant sandwiches for breakfast. Today on the kids' menu at Burger King, you'll find the basics. Their "King Jr." burgers and chicken nuggets—which is what you'll find on almost every kids' menu in America. At McDonald's, of course, you'll find their wildly famous Chicken McNugget Happy Meals on the menu. Wendy's, Arby's, and Jack in the Box all have chicken nuggets or strips on their kids' menus too. You'll also find fried chicken strips on the kids' menu at most casual restaurants like Cracker Barrel, IHOP, and even places you wouldn't normally think of serving this type of fare—Olive Garden and Red Lobster.

There's the idea out there that children won't eat unless nuggets are on the menu. Why is this? I did a little digging and found out that Burger King's Chicken Nuggets are "seasoned" with specific chemicals designed in a lab to keep you wanting to eat more: yeast extract (a hidden form of MSG) and natural flavors (which are proprietary mixtures that make food taste irresistible). You'll find similar chemicals in the chicken nuggets at Chick-fil-A, McDonald's, and Arby's. These nuggets are all fried in processed vegetable oils, breaded in white flour, and spiked with flavor enhancers to get your children hooked.

Kids' menus are filled with the most ultra-processed and sugary stuff served in the restaurant: it seems like no matter what the restaurant specializes in, kids will be offered nuggets, mac 'n' cheese, corn dogs, and the like. Does it really need to be this way? Why is there even a special menu for kids?

I am going to flip the script: you don't need to order off the kids' menu at all. I'll go more into how we dine out as a family in a moment. Let me start by saying that when children are very young, don't be afraid to bring your own food from home for them. You can prepare meals for them and take them with you into restaurants in a lunch box (or thermos or small glass jars in your diaper bag). Even if you don't bring your child's entire meal, bringing along healthy snacks (i.e., appetizers) is a great way to keep your children occupied in restaurants while waiting for courses to arrive. That way you know they are eating something nourishing and not just the French fries or chips that might be on the table.

Here's a quick list of foods that are easy to bring to restaurants:

- Steamed vegetables with butter and a little sea salt in a thermos
- Almond butter and banana sandwich on sprouted bread
- Small smoothies in a stainless steel cup or thermos with lid
- Olives
- Cheese in cubes or small slices
- Diced fruit (this makes great dessert)
- The Only Bar by Truvani (any flavor). We like to break these up into small pieces and not give our children the entire bar.

Parents often tell me they never eat at restaurants with their babies and young children. They tell me it's too much hassle to try to keep them happy and quiet, and that because they are too young to enjoy the restaurant's food, it doesn't make sense to bring them. While of course there are situations when my husband and I have a "date night" without the kids, the majority of the time we bring them with us. We love eating together as a family whenever possible. I feel that when we're eating together, they have another opportunity to learn from us. Taking your children to restaurants gives them more exposure to how you make food choices out in the world. They also learn a lot about manners to keep at the table, which we also teach at home, but it's great to practice this out in public too!

Below are my tried-and-true tips for dining out with kids. These are primarily for babies and small children; as your children grow up, these tips will evolve when they become independent eaters.

- **Place your order as soon as possible.** We never ponder the menu too long. My husband and I are in the routine of quickly looking at the menu, determining what we want, and ordering it right away with our drinks when we see the server for the first time.

- **Come prepared with some entertainment.** Bring a nice variety of sticker books, Legos, Wikki Stix, crayons, and small magnetic toys with you to help pass the time.

- **Serve your meals in courses.** This is actually how we always eat at home and this doesn't change when we are eating in a restaurant. This is a great way to keep your children occupied for the entire meal and helps them to sit for up to an hour or more. We give our children a first course that we packed for them (such as a smoothie) while we are waiting for the server to bring the first course we ordered. When our first course arrives (such as soups or salads) we give our children a second course of food that we brought with us (such as some olives). When they are older, they may eat their own salad or soup too. Then when our main dinner comes to the table, we also give them a main course, which is the stuff they really like to eat, usually the protein—turkey, black beans, or chicken. This can either be shared off our plates, or what we bring in for them in a thermos. After we all eat our main course, and if we decide to order dessert, I like to have fruit packed for the kids. Serving food in courses like this allows us more time to enjoy dining out, and we often can sit back with a glass of wine or dessert at some incredible restaurants in our hometown and while traveling.

- **Get a reusable silicone bib and suction plate.** Silicone bibs are great because you can rinse them off in two seconds. We've used disposable bibs here and there, but honestly, there is no sense in doing that when a silicone bib fits easily into a diaper bag. It also

has a little pocket that catches the food that falls, which helps keep the mess down. We couple this with a small plate with suction cups that we can attach to the table, which we use to offer each course of the meal. When I forget to bring a bib, I tie the restaurant napkin like a scarf around my baby's collar. With my second child, this happens a lot, haha.

- **Use a clip-in travel high chair.** We have a high chair from Inglesina that connects to most restaurant tables. It allows our baby to be right at the table with us and both of our children loved this. This makes it much easier for them to sit for longer periods in a restaurant as they are right there with us. It's also perfect to use while traveling and eating out more than usual.

- **Always tip extra and clean up after yourselves.** This is especially important if you bring in your own food and make any kind of mess on the floor. I always tip at least an extra 5 to 10 percent on top of my normal tip. I try to keep things tidy, of course, but I can't always be successful in keeping it all on the table (and in certain situations it is hard to completely clean up the floor on your own). I keep WaterWipes on me, which makes cleaning up the table, my children, and any other messes much easier. These are like "baby wipes," but they don't have nasty chemicals.

BIRTHDAY PARTIES

I'll never forget the time my daughter went to two different birthday parties on the same weekend when she was three. While I love kids' parties and greatly appreciate my daughter being invited to celebrate with her friends, there was something I was sad to see at both parties. The birthday cakes being served were covered in brightly colored icing that was dyed with artificial colors. Perhaps I shouldn't have been surprised. Almost every bakery in America makes their cakes with a lot of artificial colors and other shady ingredients. Have you seen the ingredients in those cakes at your grocery store bakery? The list of ingredients is a far departure from what you'd find in a traditional cake recipe primarily consisting of sugar, flour, eggs, butter, and vanilla extract. I can safely say that you'd never bake a cake at home with half of the ingredients in the supermarket version. That's because many of these ingredients are only used by the processed food industry.

Unfortunately, you'll often find the same at natural food supermarkets and bakeries. For instance, there is a grocery store near my home in Charlotte with a welcoming farmer's market vibe. It is filled with local produce and fresh flowers. I wanted to believe their in-house bakery-made cakes had fewer processed ingredients, but I did a little digging and was disappointed to find Red 40, Yellow 6, Yellow 5, and titanium dioxide added to one of their chocolate cakes. Why is this necessary? To make a chocolate cake more brown?

Take a look next time you're shopping and you'll find that most grocery store cakes are one big science experiment. While almost every ingredient in these cakes are awful, my biggest concern is that they are loaded with artificial colors. (To get the lowdown on why artificial colors are so harmful, see The Dangers of Artificial Colors on page 35.)

My close friends and family already know how detrimental artificial colors can be to children, but as my daughter attends more parties (and is now in school), her social circle is widening—and I'm seeing artificial colors everywhere. Parents accept that children need to eat these controversial dyes to celebrate birthdays because *everyone* serves birthday cake and, of course, those cakes *have to* look a certain way. It's also an accepted belief that if a child is only eating artificial colors "occasionally" at parties, it will do no harm.

And sure, for most of us adults, birthday parties are an occasional occurrence. So why should you even worry about the artificial Blue 1 on your daughter's slice of birthday cake? Because your child isn't going to one birthday party a year; they're likely going to several. And it's not just birthday parties. Your children are being bombarded with artificial colors at every turn. Everyday products specifically targeting kids are full of artificial colors, and they are being served at friends' houses and schools everywhere.

They're in children's drinks, cereals, snacks, and even "approved" school lunches.

You'll find artificial colors in just about every holiday celebration from Halloween, to Christmas, to Valentine's Day, to Easter. And then you've got the summertime backyard parties with brightly dyed Popsicles.

The point is: it's a slippery slope to allow children to eat artificial colors "just this once" or "just at this one party," because next thing you know it becomes a monthly or even weekly indulgence. And should it really be considered an indulgence? The thought of consuming artificial colors and other food-like chemicals linked to health issues on a day when we are supposed to be celebrating our life or our children's lives seems a little ironic, doesn't it? Like you, I want my children to have the best. That is why I will not compromise and allow them artificial colors at celebrations. I have a dream that someday this will be the norm.

As parents, it's our responsibility to teach our children about their food. We obviously cannot be with them their entire lives, and they will be independently exposed to many different foods over the course of their lives, so we need to teach them how to make the best choices. This is why I began teaching my children about food dyes and brightly colored treats at a very young age. I tell them what these colors are made from (petroleum) and how they are made in a factory to make food look pretty but are actually not healthy for our bodies to eat. I also teach them how to spot artificial colors in food that they're served at parties, friends' houses, schools, and restaurants. They are learning that if a cake is covered in brightly colored icing, that it is probably artificially colored and not good to eat.

Of course, I don't ever want my children to feel left out or miss out on enjoying treats. I'll suggest that they choose a white or chocolate option instead (if available) or to scrape off the colorful icing. If there are multiple treats available, let your child enjoy one of them (preferably the one without artificial colors). Also, a lot of times, my daughter is more excited about a treat I have for her in the car or in my purse, which she would rather eat than what is being served at the party. Don't feel like you need to give in to all the treats at a party.

Sometimes you may feel like your children aren't listening to you or that they're too young to understand, but you may be surprised at what they pick up. I recently arrived late to a birthday party with Harley, and all the children were eating cake when we arrived. The hostess told us that the cupcakes were made with organic ingredients without artificial dyes, but that the birthday cake from a bakery was not organic. The bakery cake also didn't have colorful frosting (so I knew it didn't have artificial dyes all over it) and looked so delicious that I really wanted to try it even though it wasn't organic. Harley chose the organic cupcake, while I helped myself to a slice of that non-organic cake I had my eye on. Harley asked me why I wasn't choosing the organic cupcake. At that moment I knew she had been paying attention to me all those times I'd been talking to her about organic food (no artificial food dyes, fewer pesticides) and why organic homemade food is what I typically like to choose. It makes me so happy to know that she has already learned so much about her food at such a young age!

LEADING BY EXAMPLE: HOW TO MAKE DELICIOUS, HEALTHY PARTY TREATS

Showing my kids how to make fun colorful treats at home without artificial colors has reinforced their love of these healthier options. And in passing down this knowledge, I hope to start a new tradition in not just my own family, but in yours too. Natural colors are inexpensive and readily available now, so it is possible to make bakery-worthy colorful treats for parties without using the artificial stuff. When Harley turned three, I made a dye-free strawberry cake and it was a big hit. I was able to make it this gorgeous shade of pink just by using crushed dried strawberries.

Here are four ingredients that will help you step up your treat game.

1. Natural Food Dyes

These may contain additives and generally are not organic, which isn't ideal; however, they are a zillion times better than artificial colors and inexpensive. Here are the best brands I've found in natural food stores and online:

- Supernatural Vegan Food Colors
- India Tree Nature's Colors Decorating Set
- Nature's Flavors Organic Food Colors

2. Freeze-Dried Fruit, Vegetable, and Spice Powders

You can use powders made out of 100 percent freeze-dried produce to dye your cakes and cookies. If you can't find the powders, you can simply buy freeze-dried fruit to make your own powder, such as strawberries, which is what I used for the Strawberry Cake recipe in my cookbook *Food Babe Kitchen*. This way your colors are also nutritious!

- Yellow: Carrot Powder, Goji Berry Powder, Goldenberry Powder
- Blue: Butterfly Pea Powder, Blue Spirulina Powder
- Pink: Dragon Fruit Powder, Freeze-Dried Strawberries, Hibiscus Powder
- Red: Beet Powder
- Purple: Purple Sweet Potato Powder, Ebony Carrot Powder, Grape Powder
- Green: Matcha Green Tea Powder, Pandan Leaf Powder, Spirulina Powder

3. Naturally Colored Sprinkles or Candies

Take a plain white cake and make it look amazing with colorful decorations.

- Let's Do Organic Confetti Sprinkelz
- Supernatural Sprinkles
- India Tree Rainbow Mix Decorating Sugar
- Unreal Milk Chocolate Gems

4. Fresh Fruit

Blend pureed berries (fresh or cooked) into cakes and frosting very easily to make them more colorful, or use chopped fruit as decoration. Since there is water in the fruit, you may need to slightly decrease the amount of liquid in your recipe.

- Strawberries
- Raspberries
- Blueberries
- Blackberries
- Pineapple
- Cherries

Do-It-Yourself Shortcuts

Don't have time to do it all yourself? Look for a bakery in your town that will bake without artificial colors. If you can't find one, ask if your local bakery will use natural colors for an extra charge; you can purchase the colors yourself or ask them to use specific brands. I've done this multiple times, and it works like a charm.

Since the frosting is typically the biggest source of artificial colors, you can also purchase plain cakes, cupcakes, and cookies, and frost them yourself. (If a ready-made plain treat isn't available, simply ask the bakery to use no dyes in the cookies or cake.)

Another option is to use organic cake mixes and organic packaged frosting. Homemade tastes best and you can totally control the ingredients you use, but if you don't want to bake from scratch you can buy mixes and make them colorful and festive with any of the options in this section. You'll find that almost every popular cake mix and frosting on the market has artificial colors added to it—including some chocolate versions. Even packaged vanilla frosting (which is white) has artificial red and yellow dye in it! This is why you want to choose a certified organic brand (which won't contain artificial ingredients) and make sure to check the ingredient list on any brand you choose. You can find the options below in natural food grocery stores or order them online to have them shipped to your house.

Dye-Free Cake Mixes

- Wholesome Organic Golden Cake Mix
- Simple Mills Vanilla Cake Mix & Chocolate Cake Mix (not organic, but real food ingredients)
- Miss Jones Organic Yellow Cake Mix & Organic Chocolate Cake Mix
- Birch Benders Organic Yellow Cake Mix & Organic Chocolate Cake Mix
- Annie's Organic Confetti Cake Mix
- Namaste Organic Yellow Cake Mix (gluten free & nut free)

Dye-Free Frosting Brands

- Simple Mills Organic Vanilla Frosting (color it any way you want!) & Chocolate Frosting

- Miss Jones Organic Buttercream Frosting, Organic Chocolate Frosting, & Birthday Buttercream Frosting

- Date Lady Organic Chocolate Spread (tastes like fudge)

I hope this gives you tons of options other than buying cakes full of artificial dyes. You can make a difference. You help to shape the marketplace when you vote with your dollars.

They say you can't have your cake and eat it too—but why not? Please share this information with your friends and family and let them know how we can all have safe, dye-free parties together!

HOLIDAY CANDY

When I was a child, I was obsessed with candy. I knew every brand, every flavor, and always had candy with me. In many childhood pictures, I'm gripping a piece of candy so that no one would take it away from me. I always found a way to have some on me, somewhere. I'd hide it in secret cabinets or in my pockets. I now know firsthand how detrimental my addiction to these "treats" were to my health, and I am so happy that I've now found a way to enjoy my life (and holidays like Halloween) without conventional candy.

When Halloween rolls around each year, I can't help but feel saddened when I see the supermarket aisles fill with gigantic bags of the very same brands I loved as a child. Year after year, it's the same traditional products—the same ones that made me so sick—along with new chemical candy creations. It seems each year candy companies are getting bolder, trying to top the competition with loads of artificial colors and additives. Do we really need "Witches Brew" Kit Kats that are dyed bright green?

I coined the phrase "Holiday Death Aisle" to describe how I feel when I see the shelves filled with toxic holiday candy filled with artificial colors, corn syrup, and artificial flavors. Many of these "festive treats" are made from the absolute worst ingredients you can put in food, and children sometimes eat these by the bucket load. Food manufacturers know they can get away with putting the cheapest ingredients in candy because they tap into the nostalgia of the holiday season. Tracey Massey, the former president of Mars Chocolate North America, even went on the record saying that Mars doesn't consider candy a food: "We're a treat. We're not a food. We're not a meal. We're a treat and consumers like to treat themselves."[2]

Parents also get sucked into the candy-buying cycle by the idea that "it's just once a year"—but, really, it's *all year*. Almost immediately after they clear the Halloween candy from their shelves, grocery stores stock up on Christmas candy. And then comes Valentine's Day. And next is Easter. It keeps going in an endless cycle of toxic seasonal treats. I'm not saying you shouldn't have festive treats for the holidays, but it baffles me how food companies and restaurants fill their holiday treats with the worst possible ingredients. Yes, I said restaurants, because they are guilty too. Have you seen what Chick-fil-A puts in their seasonal Peppermint Chip Milkshake? It's truly an abomination filled with high-fructose corn syrup, artificial colors, carrageenan, and other ultra-processed ingredients. Isn't it time we stop believing that holiday treats made with horrible ingredients are a treat?

Chick-fil-A Peppermint Chip Milkshake: Whole Milk and Nonfat Dry Milk, Sugar, Cream, Water, Contains Less Than 1% of: Whey, Mono and Diglycerides, Corn Starch, Guar Gum, Carrageenan, Calcium Sulfate, Cellulose Gum, Brown Sugar, Natural and Artificial Flavor, Natural Flavor, Salt, Caramel Color, Beta-carotene (Color), Annatto (Color), Corn Syrup, Water, Glycerin, Vegetable Juice for Color, Citric Acid, Natural Peppermint Flavor, Sodium Benzoate, Cream, Milk, Sugar, Sorbitol, Contains Less Than 2% of: Mono and Diglycerides, Carrageenan and Natural Flavor, Propellant: Nitrous Oxide, Sugar, Corn Syrup, Natural Peppermint Oil, Red 40, Confectionery Coating (Sugar, Hydrogenated Palm Kernel Oil, Cocoa [May Be Processed with Alkali], Whey Powder, Soy Lecithin [Emulsifier], Vanilla), Powdered Sugar, Corn Starch, Silicon Dioxide, Cherries, (Water, Corn Syrup, High-Fructose Corn Syrup, Citric Acid, Natural & Artificial Flavor, Potassium Sorbate, and Sodium Benzoate As Preservatives, FD&C; Red 40 and Sulfur Dioxide [Preservative]).

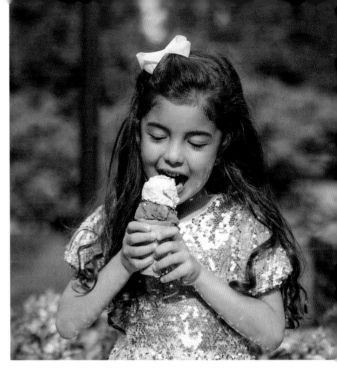

Healthy Alternatives to Seasonal Treats

Candy will never be a health food, but we can make it better—and stop relying on conventional candies to celebrate the holidays. Years ago, I switched from heavily processed holiday candies to organic brands that don't use artificial colors or other synthetic additives. Thankfully, there are some great store-bought alternatives available! I also started the tradition of making homemade holiday treats with whole food organic ingredients—and I've never looked back.

Of course, you're not going to want to make everything yourself and may need to buy packaged holiday candy. For example, if you have children in schools where homemade food is not allowed at holiday parties, you'll likely need to buy store-bought treats for candy exchanges and the like. And you know what? I too like to indulge in some candy during the holidays! I still love it, but I don't buy the toxic stuff.

First and foremost, remember to always read the ingredient list. This is the golden rule for any product, and it shouldn't be any different during the holidays. That said, when it comes to candy, I do give myself a little more leeway. Obviously every candy out there—even organic varieties—is going to have some form of sugar in it. So, while you don't need to go overboard in trying to find a "healthy candy," there are definitely some horrible ingredients that you can avoid. Let's talk about what to look out for.

Ultimate Holiday Candy Swaps List

I have a big list of holiday candy swaps for you. If you have little ones in school, many of these swaps come in wrapped individual portions, which are great for parties. While these options aren't perfect in terms of ingredients and not something I recommend eating on a regular basis (it's candy!), they are way better than conventional holiday treats, and you can find them at natural foods grocery stores or online. I typically order holiday candy online about one month before I need it.

INSTEAD OF THIS	TRY THIS
Snickers	OCHO Caramel & Peanut Bar
Hershey's Milk Chocolate	Alter Eco Truffles
Reese's Peanut Butter Cups	Justin's Peanut Butter Cups
Milky Way	Nelly's Caramel Nougat Bars
M&M's	Unreal Chocolate Gems
Mounds or Almond Joy	Nelly's Coconut Bar
Welch's Fruit Snacks	Black Forest Fruit Snacks
DumDums Pops	YumEarth Pops
Starburst	Torie & Howard Chewie Fruities
Skittles	YumEarth Giggles
Werther's Original Chewy Caramels	Cocomels Coconut Milk Caramels
Hershey's Kisses or Bars	NibMor Chocolates
Russell Stovers Assorted Chocolates	Lake Champlain Organic Boxed Chocolates
Twizzlers	YumEarth Licorice
Reese's Peanut Butter Egg	OCHO Peanut Butter Egg
Ghirardelli Squares	Lake Champlain Chocolate Squares
Brachs Candy Canes	YumEarth Candy Canes
Hershey's Chocolate Bunnies	Lake Champlain Chocolate Bunnies
Dove Promises Chocolate Caramels	OCHO Caramel Minis
York Peppermint Patties	Heavenly Organics Mint Honey Patties
Junior Mints	OCHO Peppermints
Brach's Candy Corn	YumEarth Candy Corn

Holiday Candy Ingredient Hit List

Next time you are shopping for holiday candy, use this hit list as a guide. These are some of the most common ingredients to avoid in holiday candy because they are heavily processed and may lead to health issues.

Artificial Flavors: Food companies don't need to tell you anything about the ingredients in their artificial flavors—they just slap "artificial flavors" on the ingredient label—and we are left in the dark about what we are really eating. They're usually made from cheap chemicals derived from petroleum along with solvents, emulsifiers, flavor modifiers, and preservatives.

Artificial Colors (such as Yellow 5 and Red 40): Derived from petroleum, these dyes are known to disrupt the immune system and are also linked to hyperactivity in children, which is why they require a warning label in Europe. They may be contaminated with carcinogens as well. Remember that fruit snacks are just candy too. Popular brands like Welch's artificially dye their fruit snacks with Red 40 and Blue 1 (and fill them with corn syrup, artificial flavors, and other processed ingredients). Organic fruit snacks are an okay option because they won't contain artificial ingredients or artificial colors. But don't consider fruit snacks healthy or superior to other organic candy options out there just because they have "fruit" in the name.

Titanium Dioxide: This is an artificial color added as a whitening and brightening agent. Scientists at the European Food Safety Authority (EFSA) found that it may have genotoxic effects, which means the ability to damage DNA, leading to cancer. This additive has been banned from food in Europe, but remains in U.S.-produced products.

Caramel Color: The most common form is made from ammonia and contains the chemical 4-Methylimidozale (4-MEI), which is classified as a possible carcinogen. Why add this to chocolate and caramel that should be naturally brown anyway?

Vanillin: This artificial vanilla flavor is used as a cheap alternative to vanilla extract, and is made from wood or petrochemicals.

PGPR (polyglycerol polyricinoleate): A cheap emulsifier used to replace more expensive cocoa butter.

TBHQ (tertiary butylhydroquinone): Preservative derived from petroleum that's linked to asthma, allergies, and dermatitis.

BHT (butylated hydroxytoluene): Risky preservative linked to cancer. Unnecessary and much more heavily regulated in Europe and Australia.

GMOs: Unless a candy is organic or Non-GMO Project verified, it's probably made with genetically modified (GMO) ingredients. The sugar in most conventional candy comes from GMO sugar beets or GMO corn, and if you don't see "cane sugar" on an ingredient list, that's a sign that the product contains GMO sugars. GMO sugar is sprayed with Roundup[3]—a herbicide linked to cancer and several other diseases—so it's good to avoid it at all costs. And when it comes to pesticides, the cocoa bean is one of the most heavily sprayed crops in the world, so it's very important to choose organic chocolate. Organic chocolate is also made with organic dairy, which comes from cows raised without added hormones, antibiotics, and GMO feed.

What to Do with Conventional Treats

My family has started a tradition of exchanging chemical-filled candy for a special gift. The "Switch Witch" comes the morning after Halloween and takes away all the junk if you leave it by the door and switches it out for toys, books, games, and better treats. When my child receives candy from others—either from the friendly bank teller or a loving friend that I would not purchase myself—I always read the ingredients to my child. If the item doesn't have an ingredient list, I ask if they would like an alternative instead. I have never been turned down, because my kids know that I have yummy treats waiting for them in the pantry to enjoy without controversial additives.

Remember what I said about voting with your dollars in the Birthday Parties section. Every time you make a purchase, you are sending a message. Unless we collectively vote with our dollars by choosing organic candy with better ingredients, stores are going to continue stocking their holiday shelves with "fun size" packets of additive-laden candy. Let's make a difference together, for the health of children everywhere.

TRAVELING

One of the biggest joys in my life is traveling. Now that I'm a mom, that hasn't changed—I want to travel even more so, as I want to show my children the world. I have taken a lot of trips since Harley was born. I've brought my children with me every time I've traveled. Before I had kids, I heard many parents complain about the hassles of traveling with children and how they would feel forced to feed their children processed food if they were away from home for an extended period of time. Some have focused so much on the negative, that they have chosen to not travel with their kids. I've learned to consciously drown out their voices in my head. Of course, it takes work to avoid processed food on vacation and there is extra preparation and special things you need to pack, especially when you have little ones in tow. However, it's all worth it. The joys of taking my children to see a new place with their own eyes and experience it for the first time so far outweighs any hassle. (Like my in-laws always tell me: enjoying the good things in life takes work) Watching Harley see a sea turtle (and a stingray and shark!) for the first time in the Bahamas was pretty amazing—and it was awesome for her to come home with new vocabulary because of these experiences. Her making a little fish face and expressing her excitement over what she saw—that is worth everything.

The first big trip we took with Harley was to the French West Indies for two weeks when she was about three-and-a-half months old. It was a very easy trip because her food source was on me and it was easy to breastfeed her on the plane, which helped keep her calm and happy the whole flight. Basically whenever we went to restaurants she would either breastfeed or just stay in my arms or in my wrap—she was very portable and the easiest to travel with at this age. Traveling with her became more complicated when she started eating solid foods (around 9 to 10 months). Around that time we took a work trip to L.A. together and we have made many trips since then—and so I've learned several things about what works well (and what doesn't) when we travel.

Go-To Strategies for Traveling with Kids

Create a master packing list. Make a list of everything you need on a spreadsheet, save it to your computer, and print it out every time before you take a trip. This master list, which includes everything I need to pack for my children (and myself), has saved me so much "pre-travel anxiety." I just cross out the stuff I don't need for a particular trip and start packing. I know this sounds sort of obvious, but the only thing worse than the thought of starting a packing list from scratch every time I want to go somewhere, is trying to pack without one.

Stay somewhere with a kitchen. I love using Airbnb and VRBO to find rentals that have full kitchens. This makes it easy to make breakfast, lunch, and dinner and to clean up afterward. Also, if we eat out, I can bring food I prepare in our rental to restaurants and give that to my children while we wait for our server to bring out our meals. This keeps them happy and occupied, which is another big bonus.

Pack food essentials. Pack any essentials that are hard to find elsewhere, such as organic lentil pasta, organic pasta sauce, organic green olives, sprouted quinoa, organic oats, and organic brown rice. When I have a kitchen at my destination, I can quickly cook these as soon as we arrive. I also pack sea salt, olive oil, lots of fruits and vegetables, and anything that will make my trip easier if for some reason I can't get to the grocery store right away. In terms of spices, I bring cayenne pepper for my morning lemon water and cinnamon for our oatmeal. If I'm going on a short trip, I won't bring the whole container—I'll just pour a few teaspoons in a bag or smaller glass jar.

Use Instacart or other grocery delivery services. Using one of these services saves me so much time and allows me to easily get things that are too heavy to pack or fresh fruits and veggies that I can't easily bring with me. I place my order with Insta-cart on the way from the airport to the hotel or rental, so that the food is there when we arrive. Sometimes I'll even schedule it the night before to make sure that I have glass bottled water and lemons (for our morning lemon water), and also other staples that I like to have on hand.

Pre-cook and freeze food for short trips. When Harley was a baby on solid food and we went to New York for three days, I decided to make all of her food ahead of time and freeze some of it. I used silicone con-tainers that have several different compart-ments, which allow you to freeze the perfect serving size for babies and toddlers. I froze cooked chicken, turkey, and black beans—all the things that are the basis for protein at each meal—and then all I had to cook while we were away were the vegetables to round out the meal. I used a YETI cooler that fits in my checked suitcase and keeps every-thing frozen during the entire flight—it's amazing. We had a kitchen so it was easy to make pasta, quinoa, and all the other things I needed to make. I also kept enough food in my carry-on bag for two extra meals in case we got delayed or anything like that (which does happen, so it's great to be prepared). I bring an insulated bag as a carry-on and fill it with ice after I go through airport security, or I pack a completely frozen ice pack and take that with me.

Get a mini slow cooker. In a hotel, it's easy to heat up food with a small slow cooker that fits in your checked luggage. In the morning I make oatmeal in the slow cooker, then I wash out the crockpot and put lunch in there to warm on high for 30 minutes (and the same for dinner). This also works for various other things that the kids like to eat that I can make ahead of time, such as homemade muffins and pancakes. This is extra helpful if you are staying some-where without a kitchen.

When flying, bring more than one meal with you. Don't just bring lunch if you plan to be flying during lunchtime. Bring lunch, din-ner, and snacks, just in case you get stuck for longer than anticipated. For example, on the way back home from the Bahamas we were delayed five hours, and so Harley had to eat lunch at the airport and dinner on the flight, as we ended up traveling all day.

Bring a travel high chair. We love that awesome Inglesina high chair I mentioned earlier that connects to most tables and is so fabulous. At restaurants, I love to use this with a little plate that suctions to the table. I'll also bring WaterWipes with me to clean it off. We started packing our travel high chair in the stroller and it's been really awesome because it allows our baby to be right at the table with us, no matter what the table height is. Both of our children loved it and would sit for at least an hour at a time for each meal—breakfast, lunch, and dinner—while we enjoyed different restaurants.

Be flexible and don't worry about making sacrifices. Depending upon where you travel, you won't always find organic food. Generally when traveling within the U.S. I am able to buy all organic because it's readily available—but when I travel internationally, I often have to make some exceptions. For instance, when staying in the Bahamas we found literally nothing organic except milk. However, fresh fruit and vegetables were readily available. So I bought broccoli because it's one of our favorite things to eat, and some other non-organic fruits and vegetables, which was much better than resorting to processed food. That's what you do when you travel—you have to understand that not everything will be organic and not get stressed out about it. I know that our diet is clean at home when we do have the choice, and that is how we set our children up for a really healthy life. The human body is resilient, and again, it is your habits, routines, and how you spend the majority of your time that really matters in the long run. You can say I looked the other way, but I understand there is balance in this life, and I never want my children to grow up feeling like their choices (and travels) are limited based on my ideas about what we should be buying. I want to be flexible in the way I raise them. If there's one thing I've learned, it's that trying to always eat 100 percent organic while traveling would make me go crazy. I've had to remind myself over and over again that the joys and experience of travel outweigh eating organic while we're

there, which relaxes my anxious mind. When I'm in control and have the choice, I'll choose organic. But if I don't have the choice, then I'll make sacrifices. The same goes for naps. I know Finley will be perfectly fine if he misses a nap and gets a little off his normal routine. During travel delays and other unexpected situations, my children always surprise me. They are both little troopers!

Stay at hotel chains that offer amenities to children. By far the best experiences we've had traveling have been when we stayed at hotels that catered to children. Even fancy ones like the Four Seasons have the most amazing kid-friendly amenities. We spent a week one summer at the Four Seasons Jackson Hole, and that experience was magical for Harley. The Four Seasons welcomed her with her own set of toys, a cute stuffed moose, and snacks in our hotel room when we arrived. They even outfitted her with her own cute robe. Breakfast was free for her—which was awesome, because it was a ridiculous buffet that had bowls and bowls of whole fruit that we could stash to eat later in the day. Even the kids' menu had healthy options, like salmon with broccoli and rice. It felt like a true vacation for me, since I didn't have to cook every meal and I could trust the restaurant to make healthy and nutritious meals for Harley.

I hope this inspires you to travel with your children if you aren't doing so already, no matter what age they are. What are you waiting for? Bon Voyage!

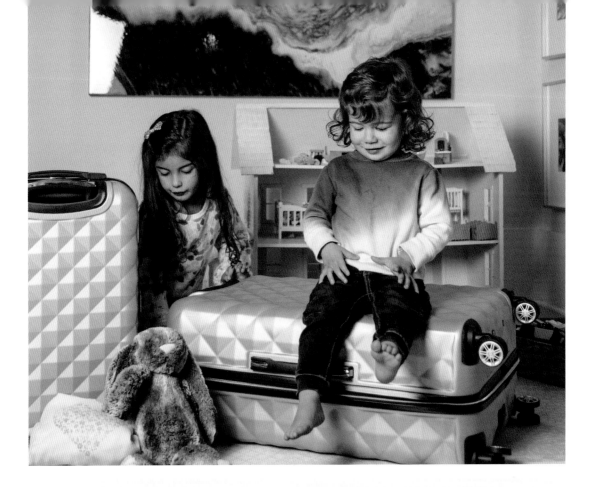

Essentials to Pack When Traveling with Young Children

- Utensils (small spoons and forks)
- Stainless steel lunch box
- Silicone plate
- Stainless steel cups with silicone lids
- Thermos
- Silicone bib
- Silicone cups for snacks
- Stainless steel bowls
- Freezer compartment containers
- 4-ounce jars to store food

- Plastic containers to store food (I normally use glass but make this exception for traveling. It makes sense because it's less weight.)
- Hot water kettle
- Mini slow cooker
- Travel high chair
- YETI cooler that can fit in a suitcase (amazing at keeping food cold for long flights)
- Insulated lunch bag

EVENTS, SHOWS, AND CONCERTS

When Harley was two, we took her to her first live musical—*Daniel Tiger Live*—and it was such a fun experience! We have pretty strict rules about screen time at my house, which has gotten more lax as she has gotten older. During potty training, I started sharing some Daniel Tiger videos to help her grasp the concepts of how it all goes down, and it turns out that Daniel Tiger has several cute videos and educational episodes. So I've allowed her to watch those while traveling on long car or plane rides. Seeing *Daniel Tiger Live* was pretty much the biggest deal in the world to her at the time. It was pretty cute to see how excited she was. Even after two hours of sitting and watching the show she wanted even more after we left.

You might be wondering what this has to do with food or why I'm even telling you this story. The reason I'm sharing this is because *Daniel Tiger Live* started at 5:30 P.M., which is dinner time at our house. I decided that instead of missing dinner, snacking at the show, and then having a late dinner and consequently a late bedtime, I would feed Harley dinner early at 4 P.M. This worked really well: she ate her normal dinner so that she was already really full when we got to the show, and she didn't need to snack for the first hour of it. But around us, we saw a totally different story.

If you have ever taken your kids to a children's musical or live event like this you have probably seen all of the concessions full of junk food snacks. I literally couldn't count the number of people eating Dippin' Dots,

Skittles, Rice Krispy Treats, and Cheez-Its. Unfortunately these snacks are all riddled with ingredients that my children never eat (and I don't eat them either), such as artificial colors.

I know that parents were simply buying what was available at the event, and it was so disappointing that there were zero healthier options. Some parents, like me, must have brought in their own snacks, but a lot of the excitement of going to shows like this is buying the "treats" that are offered.

I sat there feeling like an alien. There we were, snacking on raisins that I packed in my bag, while everyone around us was snacking on junk food. Thankfully, my daughter sat there happily eating her raisins (which are one of her favorite snacks) and didn't notice that what we were eating was any different than those around us. Of course, I want my children to fit in and eat what everyone else is eating, but that doesn't mean that I have to buy snacks made with controversial food additives linked to so many health risks. My children don't live in a bubble. I hope to take them to several more live shows and events like this, and they both will eventually be in school where they will be exposed daily to various junk foods and processed fast foods served there. I've heard this just gets worse as they get older, as many parents have described to me.

This got me thinking. What can we do as parents to have options for children at these events that are healthier? Wouldn't it be great if there was a fruit cart with little containers of blueberries, strawberries, bananas, and oranges? What if that fruit cart

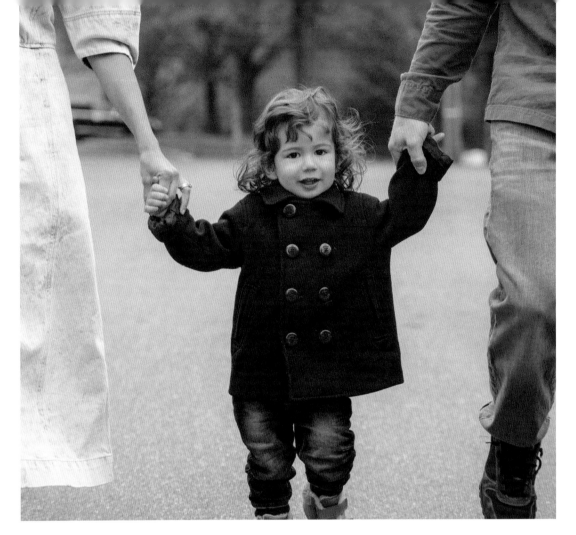

was there instead of a Dippin' Dots cart? Can we do something so that we can protect the next generation? Perhaps we can start small and influence change at one event space at a time, but I know it's a long time coming. Until then, the best thing we can do is provide our children better options.

If you want to keep buying the Cheez-Its, Lays, Skittles, and Dippin' Dots when you go to events, go right ahead. I'm not here to preach at anyone. I'm sharing my experience with you to bust the myth that this is

necessary and to give you some healthier options. Next time you take your child to an event where you know unhealthy snacks will be served, here are some tips:

- **Eat dinner or lunch earlier and right before the show.** This way your children (and you) won't be hungry and overly tempted to eat the sugary junk food from the concession stands. Feel free to rearrange your schedule a little bit to accommodate.

- **Have a parking lot picnic before you go in**. One beautiful thing we saw on our way into Daniel Tiger was a family having a picnic in the back of their car in the parking lot, with the trunk open, eating bananas and cheese sticks. I thought it was a fun idea to have a little picnic before you go into the show. Kudos to that mom because my daughter wanted to join the picnic as well!

- **Pack a few of your own snacks to bring inside**. Of course it's fun to snack during events, so make sure you're prepared. I have had no issues bringing in my own snacks. I've heard that some events don't technically allow for this, but honestly, I would pack snacks anyway. If they question it, you can let them know that your child is on a special diet, which is the truth if the food being served there isn't something that they eat. As my children are on an organic unprocessed diet, and those options are not available there, I'm being completely honest.

Snack Ideas for Events

Pack one or two of these in your bag per child:

- Any type of raw fruit in a little jar
- Bananas
- Truvani's The Only Bar
- Cheese
- Raisins
- Dried fruit
- Freeze-dried fruit
- Organic spelt pretzels
- Smoothies in a silicone pouch or thermos

Okay, friends, now it's time to implement everything you've learned in this book so far. Let's get into the kitchen and cook with some delicious real food. In the next chapters, you'll find over 100 of my family's favorite recipes. This is what we regularly eat for breakfast, lunch, dinner, and everything in between. I've also included a section on lunch boxes, which breaks down exactly what you'll often find in my daughter's school lunches.

From my family to yours, we congratulate you on going on this real food journey with us. It may not always be an easy road, but I promise that as you cook and eat real food together, you are creating incredible memories that your children will never forget. There is no greater gift.

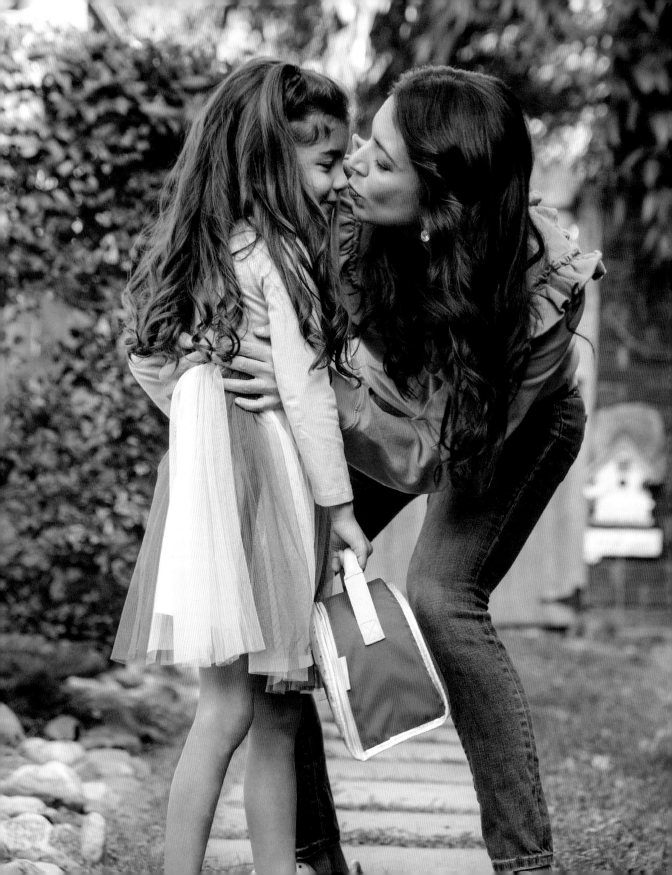

EAT LIKE A FOOD BABE FAMILY

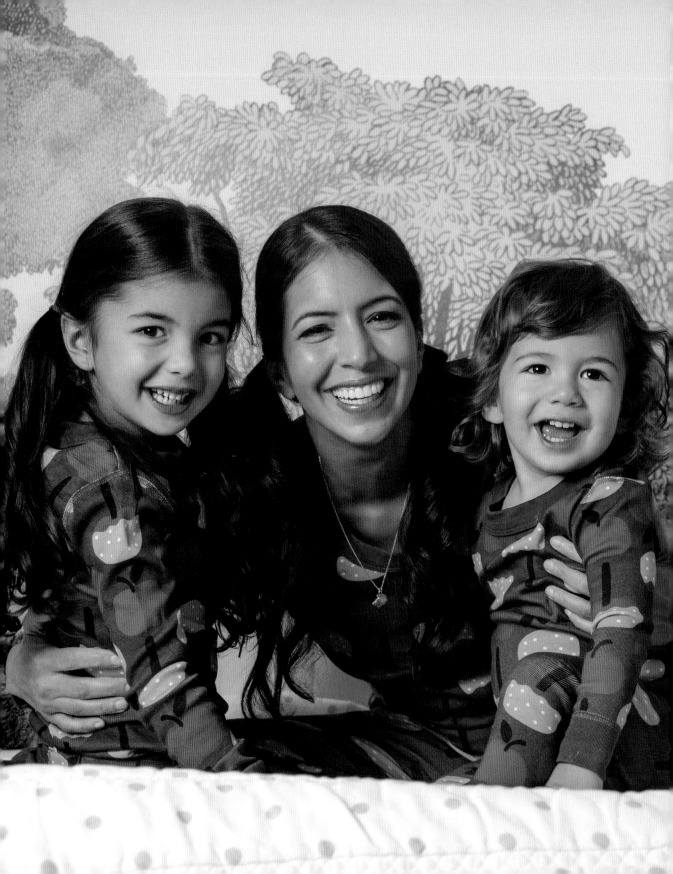

chapter 5

BREAKFAST

FUN WITH SHAPES FRENCH TOAST

Harley loves French toast, and it's even better when it's in cute shapes. I use cookie cutters to make hearts, stars, and animal cutouts. We have fun decorating them together with blueberries, strawberries, banana slices, and various other toppings. Also, Harley goes gaga for mini French toast made out of leftover slices of sourdough baguette. No cookie cutter required!

Makes 4 servings
Prep Time: 10 minutes
Cook Time: 10 minutes
Total Time: 20 minutes

1 cup almond milk or milk of choice

2 eggs

1 ripe banana, peeled

1 tablespoon coconut sugar

1 tablespoon vanilla extract

1 teaspoon ground cinnamon

Pinch of sea salt

1 teaspoon grass-fed butter

8 to 10 slices sourdough bread or bread of choice

1 tablespoon pure maple syrup (optional)

Place all ingredients except the butter, bread, and maple syrup in a blender and blend until well combined.

Arrange the bread slices in a large baking dish and pour the liquid mixture over them. Let the bread soak for at least 3 minutes per side.

Heat 1 teaspoon of butter on a griddle or skillet over medium heat. Add the soaked bread slices and cook them for 2 to 3 minutes per side or until they are golden brown.

If you are making shapes with the bread, use a cookie cutter to cut out desired shapes. Serve with desired toppings or maple syrup.

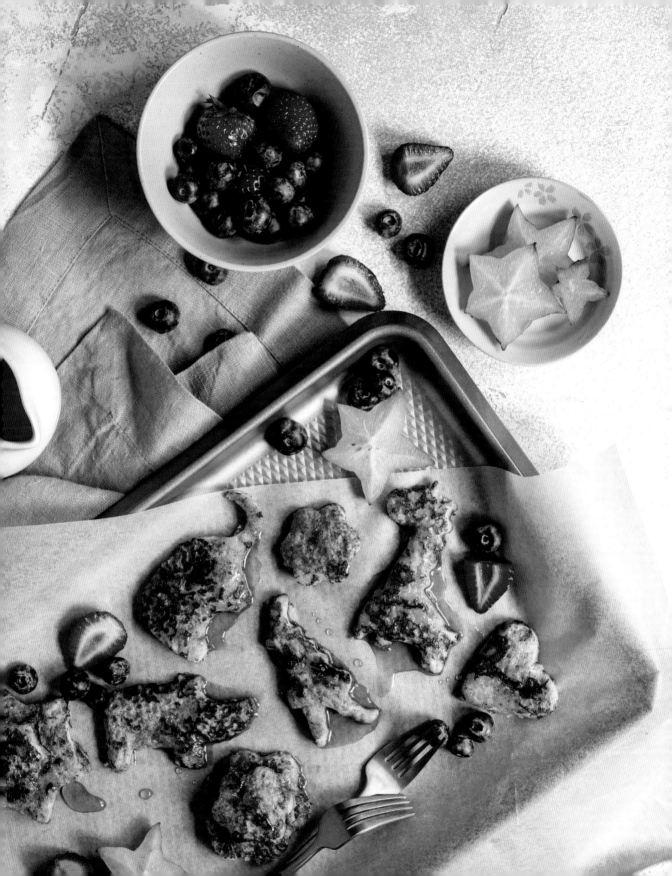

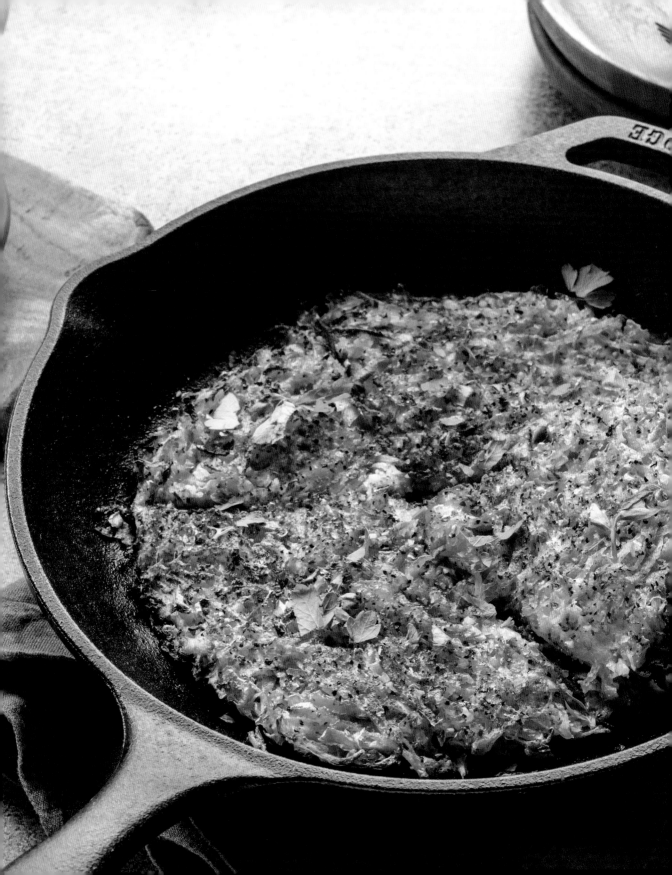

CAULIFLOWER POTATO HASH BROWNS

I always try to include vegetables with breakfast (and every meal), and this is one way I do it. We sneak some healthy cauliflower into these hash browns, and you'd never know it! These are delicious with a fried egg on top. Add an avocado too for some healthy fats.

Makes 2 to 4 servings
Prep Time: 15 minutes
Cook Time: 12 minutes
Total Time: 27 minutes

2 medium Yukon Gold potatoes (7 to 8 ounces each)
1 cup freshly grated cauliflower
½ teaspoon sea salt
¼ teaspoon ground black pepper
¼ teaspoon paprika
2 to 3 tablespoons olive oil
½ cup minced yellow onion
1 garlic clove, minced

Peel the potatoes, then grate them using the large holes on a box grater (you should have about 3 cups of shredded potatoes). Using a clean, dry dish towel, firmly twist and squeeze as much liquid as possible from the potatoes until they are very dry (you should have about 2 cups when finished).

Place the shredded potatoes in a bowl and mix in the cauliflower, salt, pepper, and paprika. Set aside.

Heat the oil in a 12-inch cast-iron skillet over medium-high heat. Add the onion and garlic and sauté for 2 minutes. Add the grated potato mixture and spread it evenly in the pan, roughly ¼ inch thick. Cook the potatoes until they are golden brown on bottom, about 5 minutes (do not disturb the potatoes or press down on them while cooking).

Use a large spatula to flip the potatoes over in one big piece (or flip them over in several sections if easier). Cook them until they are golden brown on bottom, about 4 minutes.

EASY AVOCADO TOAST

You can make this simple avocado toast in the morning in a FLASH. But to make it more fun, I like to add a cute toothpick or cut the toast into a shape using a cookie cutter. If I have them, I will sprinkle pomegranate seeds on top for the kids and red pepper flakes for the adults—that way it almost looks like we are eating the same thing, haha!

Makes 2 servings
Prep Time: 5 minutes

1 avocado, peeled and pitted
½ small lemon, juiced
Sea salt and ground black pepper to taste
2 slices toasted sprouted-grain bread
Pomegranate seeds (optional)
Sprinkle of red pepper flakes, for the adults (optional)

In a bowl, mash together the avocado, lemon juice, salt, and pepper.

To serve, spread the avocado mix on each slice of toast. Sprinkle the toast with pomegranate seeds or red pepper flakes or an additional topping of your choice, if desired.

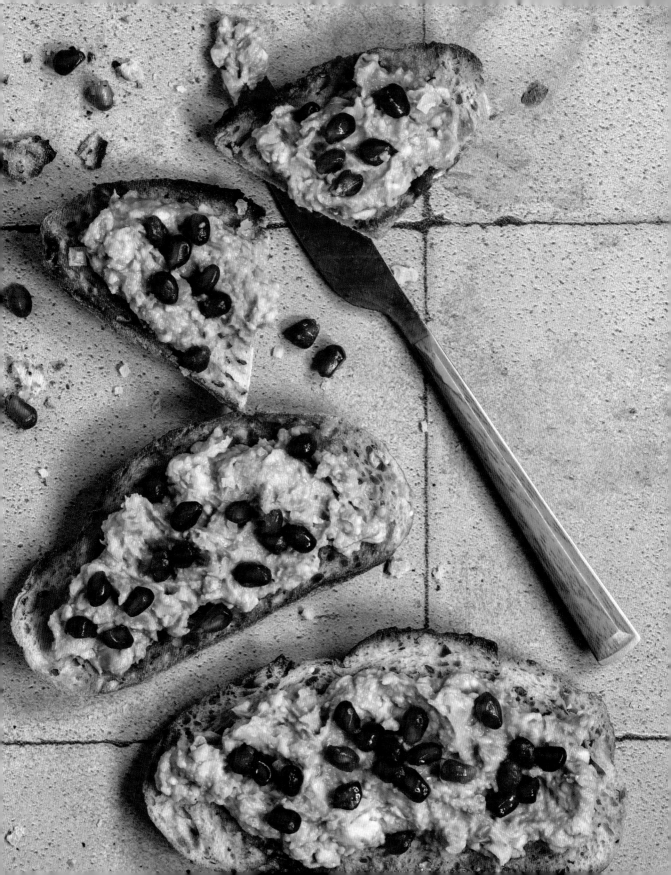

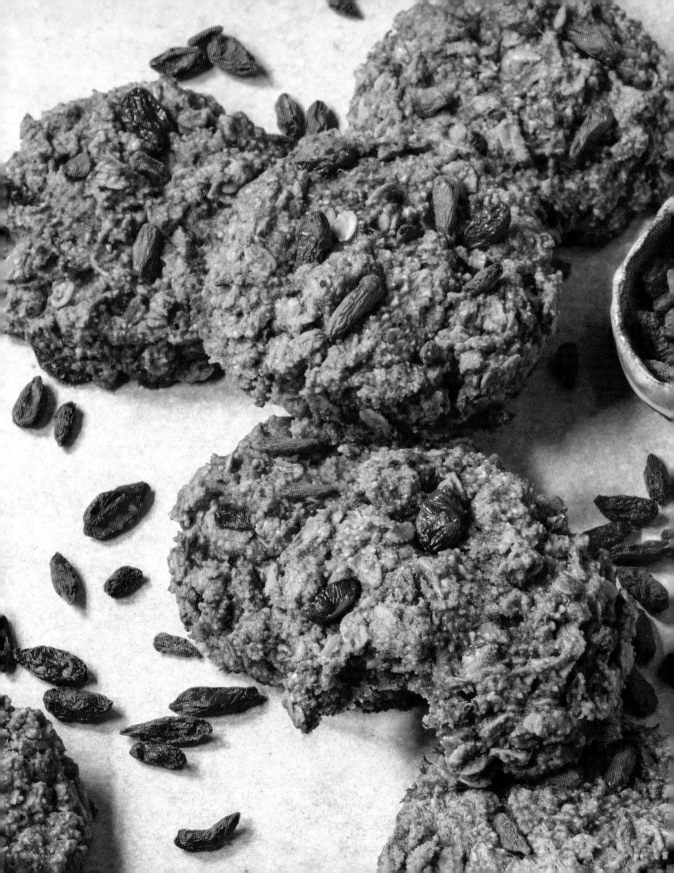

GOJI BERRY
BREAKFAST COOKIES

Who says you can't eat cookies for breakfast? Instead of white flour and white refined sugar, these cookies are made with nutrient-dense oats and almond flour. And instead of processed white sugar, they're sweetened with ripe bananas, a touch of unrefined organic coconut sugar, and chewy goji berries. Dig in!

Makes 8 to 10 cookies
Prep Time: 15 minutes
Cook Time: 15 to 17 minutes
Total Time: 30 to 32 minutes

1 ¼ cups almond flour
1 cup rolled oats
2 tablespoons ground flaxseed
1 teaspoon ground cinnamon
1 teaspoon baking soda
½ teaspoon sea salt
1 egg
⅓ cup coconut sugar
2 large ripe bananas, peeled and mashed
1 ½ teaspoons vanilla extract
¼ cup melted coconut oil
¼ cup goji berries

Preheat the oven to 375°F.

Whisk together the almond flour, oats, flaxseed, cinnamon, baking soda, and salt in a large bowl.

In a separate bowl, whisk together the egg, coconut sugar, mashed bananas, vanilla, and coconut oil.

Mix the dry ingredients into the wet ingredients. Fold in the goji berries.

Shape the mixture into 8 to 10 soft balls. Place them on a parchment-lined baking sheet, spacing them roughly 2 inches apart. Using your fingertips, gently flatten each cookie to a 2 ½- to 3-inch round.

Bake until golden brown, 15 to 17 minutes. Transfer the cookies to a wire rack to cool. You can store them in an airtight container for up to 4 days.

BERRYLICIOUS BAKED OATMEAL

with Coconut Almond Streusel

This delicious baked oatmeal is something I love to serve on lazy, rainy weekend mornings. It fills our home with the most amazing smell of warm cinnamon. So comforting!

Makes 4 to 6 servings
Prep Time: 15 minutes
Cook Time: 40 to 45 minutes
Total Time: 55 to 60 minutes

BERRYLICOUS BAKED OATMEAL

1½ cups almond milk or milk of choice

1 egg

1 ripe banana, peeled and mashed (½ to ⅔ cup)

¼ cup pure maple syrup

1 teaspoon baking powder

1 teaspoon ground cinnamon

1 teaspoon vanilla extract

½ teaspoon sea salt

2 ½ cups rolled oats

2 cups mixed berries

COCONUT ALMOND STREUSEL

1 cup unsweetened coconut flakes

½ cup sliced raw almonds

½ teaspoon ground cinnamon

½ teaspoon vanilla extract

2 tablespoons unrefined virgin coconut oil, melted

Preheat the oven to 350°F.

To make the oatmeal: Whisk together the milk, egg, banana, syrup, baking powder, cinnamon, vanilla, and salt in a large mixing bowl. Mix in the oats, then fold in the berries.

To make the streusel: Mix all the ingredients in a small bowl.

Pour the oatmeal mixture into a parchment-lined 9 x 9-inch baking pan. Top the oatmeal with the streusel and bake until a toothpick inserted in the middle comes out clean (40 to 45 minutes). Serve warm.

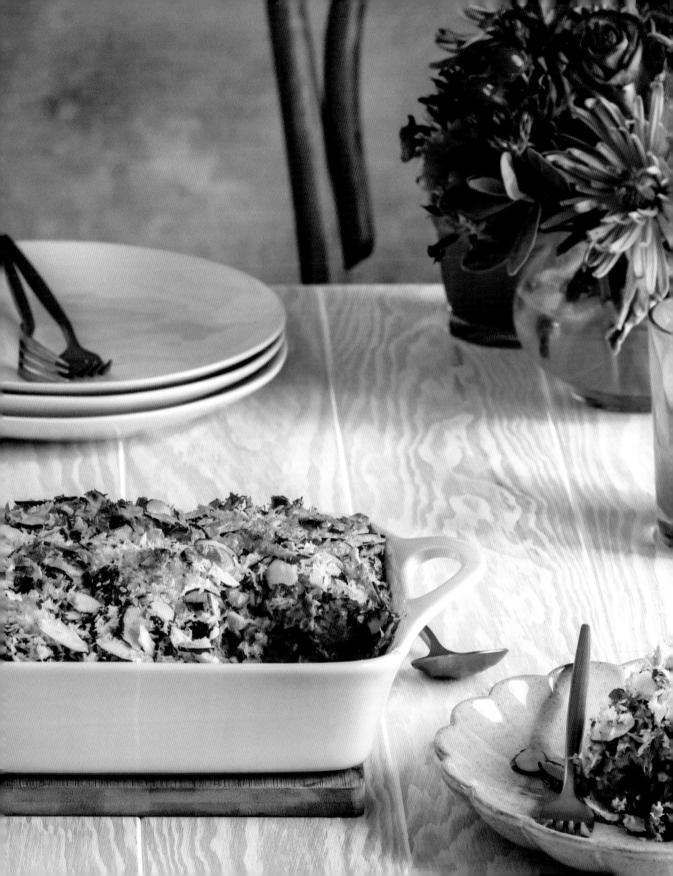

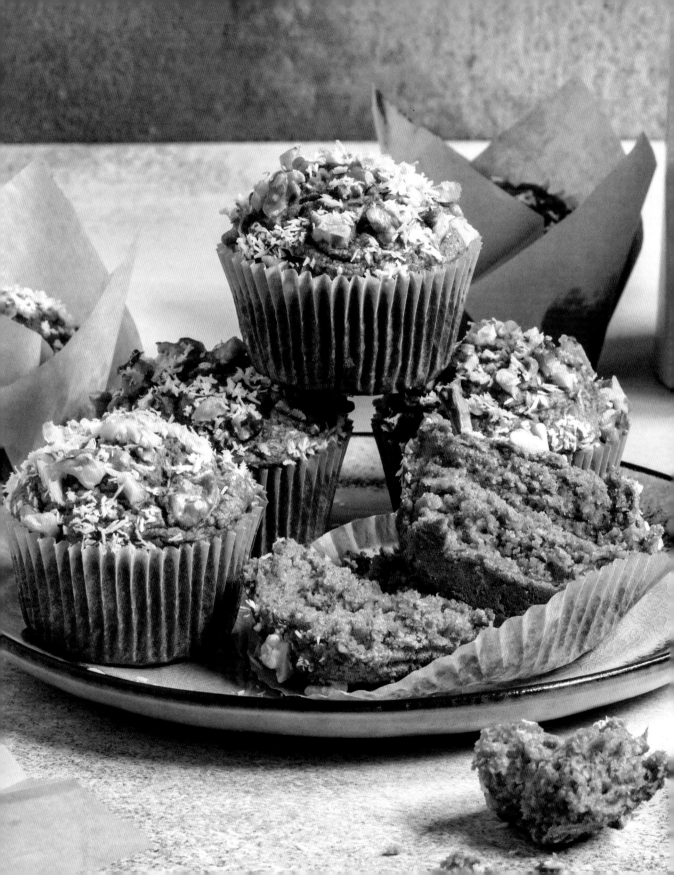

CARROT CAKE MUFFINS

These muffins are a wonderful treat at breakfast, and they're perfect to pack for a healthy on-the-go snack. They're gluten-free and have no added refined sugar, but are super moist and delicious. When I can, I'll freeze part of a batch so that we have them on hand for busy mornings—but they usually don't last long in my house!

Makes 10 to 12 muffins
Prep Time: 15 minutes
Cook Time: 22 to 25 minutes
Total Time: 37 to 40 minutes

1 ½ cups oat flour
1 cup almond flour
1 ½ teaspoons ground cinnamon
1 teaspoon baking soda
1 teaspoon baking powder
½ teaspoon sea salt
1 egg
¾ cup almond milk or canned coconut milk
1 ripe banana, peeled and mashed (½ to ⅔ cup)
½ cup pure maple syrup
1 ½ teaspoons vanilla extract
1 cup grated carrots

Optional Toppings

Shredded unsweetened coconut or coconut flakes

Chopped raw nuts

Preheat the oven to 350°F.

Whisk together the dry ingredients in a large bowl.

In a separate bowl, whisk together the egg, milk, banana, syrup, and vanilla.

Pour the wet ingredients into the dry ingredients and mix gently until combined. Fold in the carrots.

Line a cupcake pan with liners or grease with coconut oil and fill each cup until ¾ full. Sprinkle with your toppings of choice, if using. Bake until a toothpick inserted in the center comes out clean, about 22 to 25 minutes. Transfer the muffins to a rack to cool.

CHIA SEED FRUIT SALAD

I love to eat fruit in the morning—it's so energizing! This fruit salad is so heavenly that I sometimes serve it for dessert, but it's also so healthy that it can be served with any meal. It contains zero refined sugar and is full of wonderful chia seeds, which are incredibly filling and packed with health-boosting benefits!

Makes 4 to 6 servings
Prep Time: 10 minutes, plus at least 30 minutes to chill

4 cups of diced fresh fruit of choice
¼ cup currants, raisins, or goji berries
2 cups almond or coconut milk
⅓ cup chia seeds
Zest of one orange
Juice of one orange
1 tablespoon vanilla extract
¼ teaspoon ground cinnamon
½ cup shredded coconut
Handful of mint leaves

In 4 dessert bowls, add 1 cup diced fruit to each and top with 1 tablespoon of currants, raisins, or goji berries.

In a mixing bowl, combine the milk, chia seeds, orange zest, orange juice, vanilla, and cinnamon. Pour ½ cup of the mixture over the fruit in each bowl. Top with shredded coconut.

Refrigerate for at least 30 minutes (or overnight). To serve, add a few mint leaves to each bowl.

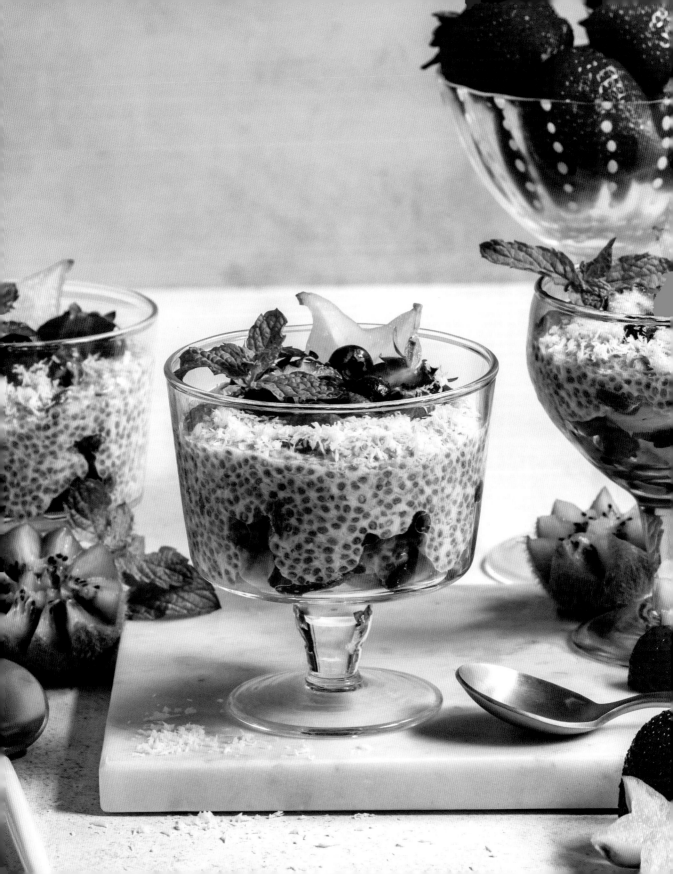

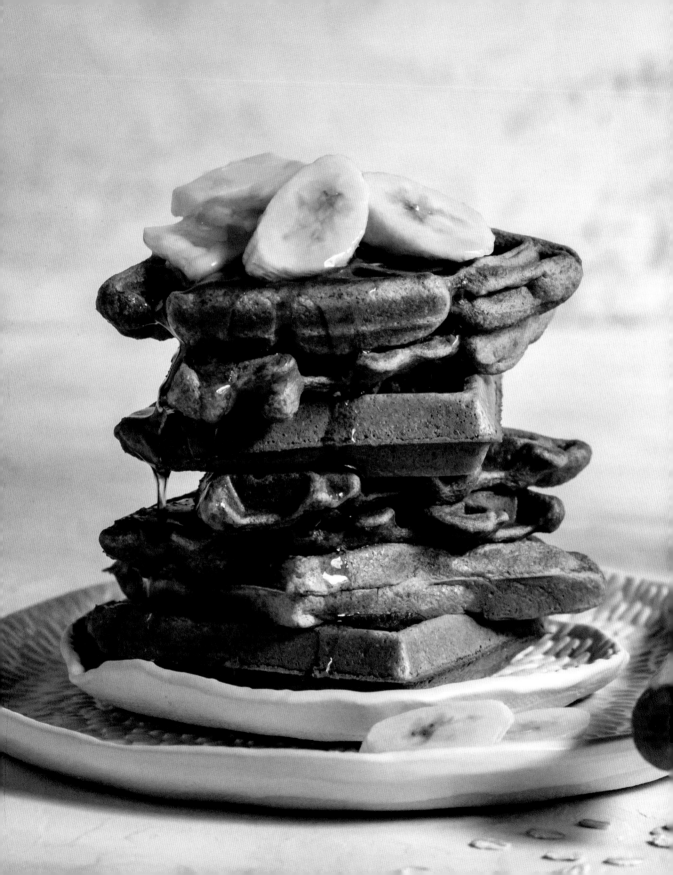

FAST GREEN WAFFLES

Instead of buying those artificially dyed frozen waffles in grocery stores, try these fun green waffles. You can make a big batch on the weekend and freeze them between sheets of parchment paper to reheat later in the toaster. They'll make your child feel like a superhero—full of energizing spinach and protein to start their day off right.

Makes 4 servings
Prep Time: 5 minutes
Cook Time: 15 minutes
Total Time: 20 minutes

1 ½ cups oat flour

2 ½ tablespoons coconut sugar

1 tablespoon baking powder

½ teaspoon ground cinnamon

½ teaspoon sea salt

2 cups loosely packed spinach

1 ripe banana

⅔ cup coconut milk

2 eggs

2 tablespoons melted coconut oil

4 tablespoons maple syrup, for serving

Preheat and grease a waffle iron.

In a bowl, mix together the flour, sugar, baking powder, cinnamon, and salt.

Place the spinach, banana, coconut milk, eggs, and oil in a blender and blend until combined. Pour into the bowl with the dry ingredients and stir to combine.

Spoon roughly ¼ cup batter onto a hot waffle iron. Cook until golden brown or until the timer goes off, about 4 minutes.

Serve the waffles hot with a dash of pure maple syrup or grass-fed butter.

SWEET POTATO AND TURKEY FRITTATA

This delicious breakfast includes one of my all-time favorite vegetables. Sweet potatoes are rich in beta carotene—a potent antioxidant—along with lutein, which make them fantastic for your eyes and vision. If you haven't tried a sweet potato with your eggs before, you are in for a real treat. There's something about these two together that is really fabulous. If you want to make a vegetarian version, just substitute 2 cups of chopped kale for the turkey.

Makes 4 to 6 servings
Prep Time: 10 minutes
Cook Time: 20 minutes
Total Time: 30 minutes

1 tablespoon unrefined virgin coconut or olive oil

8 ounces ground turkey

1 cup diced sweet potato

6 eggs

1 teaspoon chili powder

½ teaspoon sea salt

¼ teaspoon ground black pepper

¼ cup chopped fresh parsley

Preheat the oven to 400°F.

Heat the oil in a 10-inch oven-safe skillet over medium-high heat. Add the turkey and sauté until it is no longer pink, about 5 minutes. Add the sweet potato to the skillet with the turkey; cover the skillet and cook until the sweet potato is just tender, adding water to the pan by tablespoonfuls if dry, about 5 minutes. Use a metal spatula to stir and scrape up any browned bits from the bottom of the pan.

In a bowl, whisk the eggs, chili powder, salt, and pepper. Pour the egg mixture over the sweet potatoes and turkey and place the skillet in the oven. Bake until the frittata is firm and set, about 10 minutes.

Cut the frittata into wedges while it's in the skillet and transfer the wedges to plates. Sprinkle with parsley and serve.

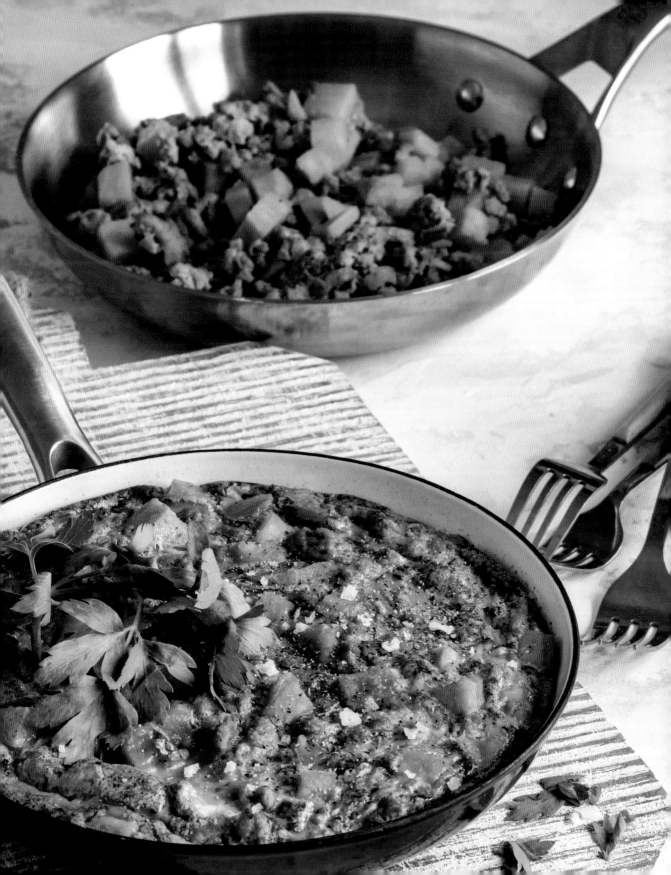

ON-THE-GO PROTEIN OATMEAL JARS

Instead of starting your day with a sugary pro-cessed breakfast that will put you in a food coma, try these easy-to-make Protein Oatmeal Jars. They will fill you up with nutrients to keep you focused and ready for the day. This is the perfect recipe to prepare ahead of time: make a few jars in the evening so they'll be ready to go on busy mornings.

Makes 1 serving
Prep Time: 5 minutes

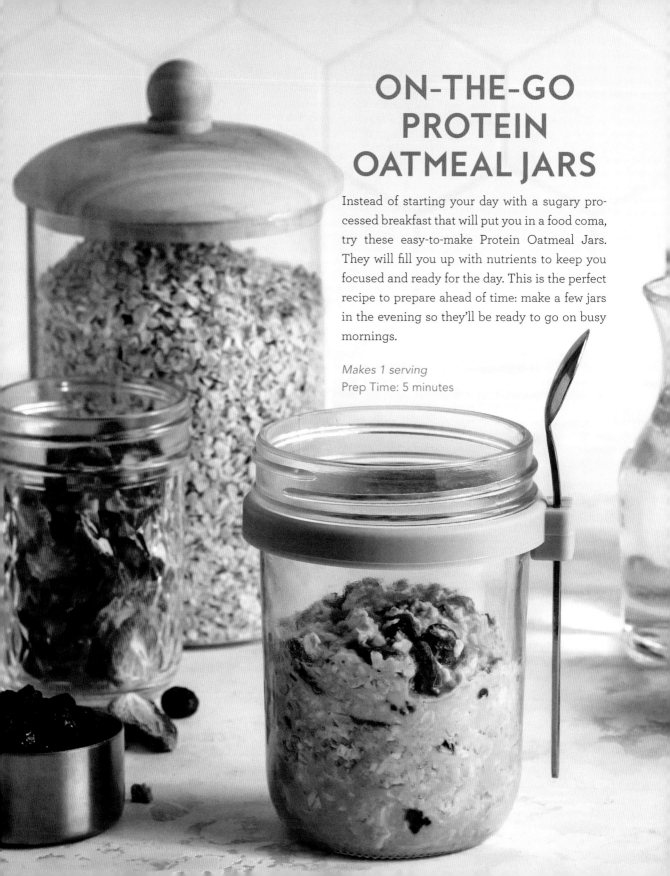

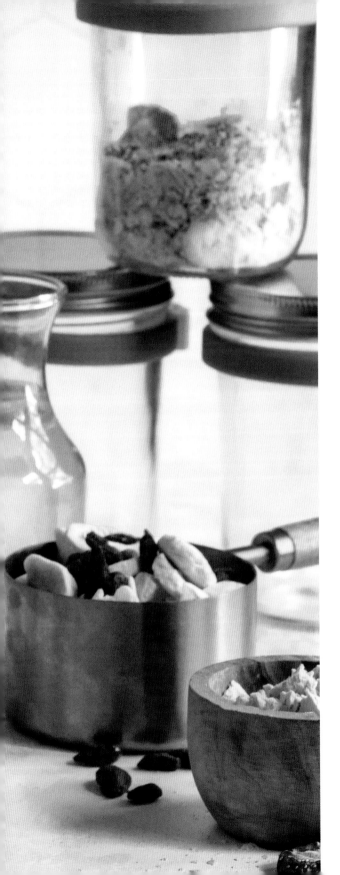

½ cup rolled oats

½ scoop Truvani protein powder (optional)

½ teaspoon ground cinnamon

¼ cup dried fruit of choice

2 tablespoons slivered almonds

Pinch of sea salt

1 cup almond milk or milk of choice (optional)

Place all the ingredients in a to-go jar and shake to combine.

When you're ready to eat, pour 1 cup of hot water in the jar and let it sit for at least 5 minutes. Alternatively, you can add almond milk to the jar instead of water and refrigerate it overnight for "overnight oats."

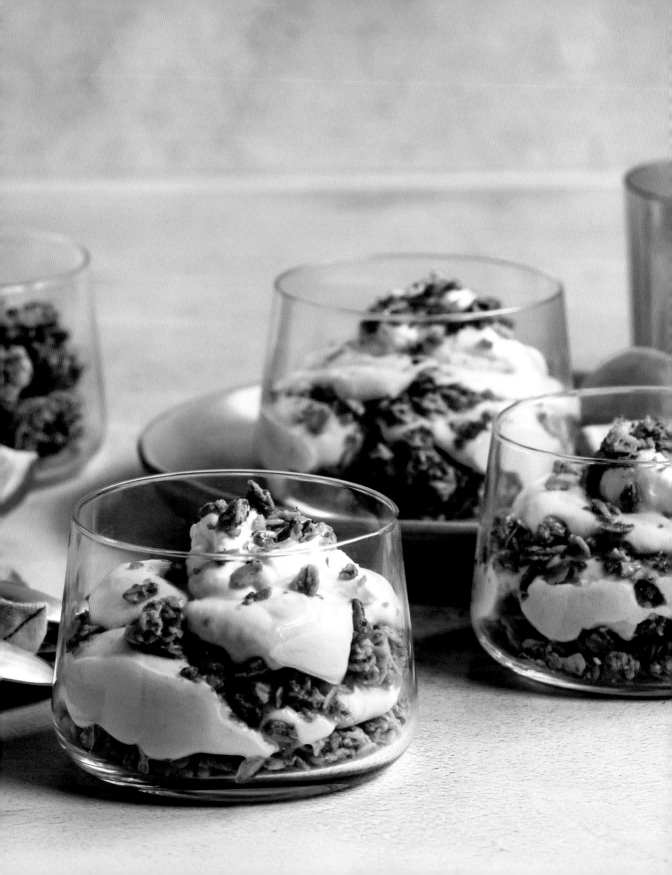

KEY LIME PIE PARFAIT

If you're stuck in a rut eating the same old oatmeal, yogurt, or eggs for breakfast, you can shake things up with this ridiculously delicious parfait. It's creamy, tart, and full of fiber and nutrients that will keep you satisfied all morning long. These parfaits also make a yummy cool summer treat.

Makes 4 servings
Prep Time: 10 minutes

2 large avocados (about 7 ounces each), peeled and pitted

¾ cup canned coconut milk

2 limes, zested and juiced

3 to 4 tablespoons raw honey

⅛ teaspoon sea salt

2 cups granola of choice

Place all the ingredients except the granola in a blender and blend until smooth (a mousse-like consistency).

Add ¼ cup granola to a short glass or cup and top it with a scant ¼ cup of the key lime pie mousse. Repeat the granola and mousse layers once more and serve.

FINLEY'S EGGS IN A BASKET

The novelty of this recipe never wears off, and you can make it even more fun by using different cookie cutters. My husband, Finley, loves making this for our daughter—who loves the crispy edges filled with buttery goodness. It's a sure way we can get her to eat some eggs even though she doesn't usually prefer them.

Makes 4 servings
Prep Time: 5 minutes
Cook Time: 5 minutes
Total Time: 10 minutes

4 slices of sourdough bread
1 teaspoon grass-fed butter
4 eggs
Sea salt and ground black pepper to taste

Cut a shape in the middle of each slice of bread. A heart or star is always fun for kids.

Melt the butter in a sauté pan over medium heat. Add a slice of bread to the pan. Crack an egg into the middle of the shape. Season with salt and pepper. Cook for about 2 to 3 minutes per side and serve.

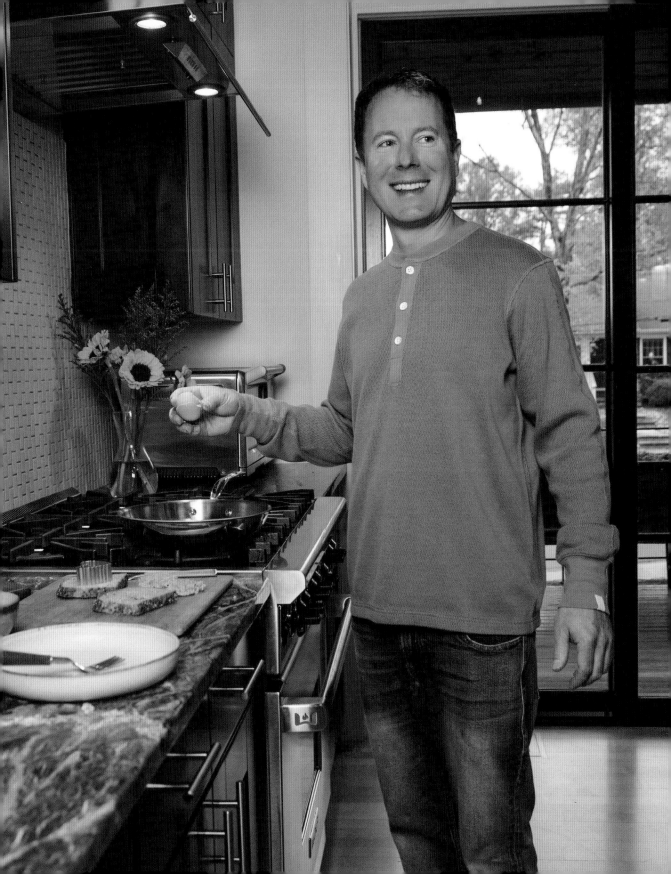

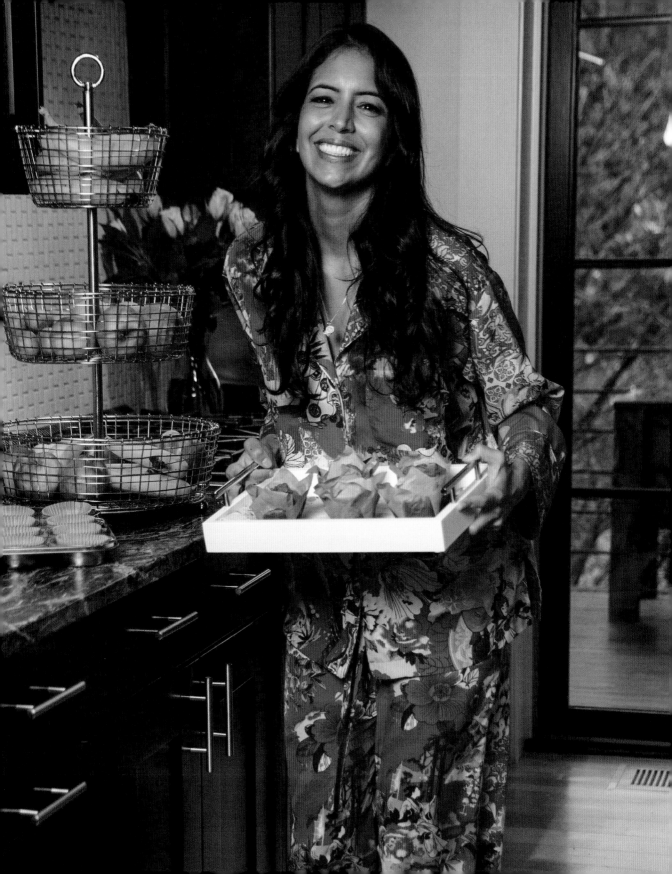

PUMPKIN MUFFINS

I love switching up the type of muffins I serve my kids. I want them to enjoy a variety of fruits and vegetables, and I love how good pumpkin is for them and me. These pumpkin muffins are perfect for freezing and reheating on busy school mornings. They also are a great lunch box addition.

Makes 10 to 12 muffins
Prep Time: 5 minutes
Cook Time: 20 to 22 minutes
Total Time: 25 to 27 minutes

½ 15-ounce can pumpkin puree
1 ripe banana, peeled
2 eggs
⅓ cup coconut oil
¼ cup raw honey or pure maple syrup
1 teaspoon vanilla extract
2 cups rolled oats
1 teaspoon baking soda
¼ teaspoon baking powder
½ teaspoon sea salt
½ teaspoon pumpkin pie spice

Preheat the oven to 350°F.

Place all the ingredients in a blender and blend until well combined. If making a vegan version of this recipe, substitute 2 tablespoons ground flaxseed mixed with 6 tablespoons of water for the eggs.

Pour the batter into a lined muffin tin; each cup should be ¾ full. Bake for 20 to 22 minutes or until a toothpick inserted in the center comes out clean.

MUESLI

I came up with this recipe after a vacation at a resort in Mexico. I ate something similar every morning, and when we got home, I knew I needed to re-create it. I e-mailed the hotel to ask for the recipe and found out the one I had been eating had so much added sugar! I knew I could come up with something just as tasty but without the sugar load—and I sure did. This muesli is awesome.

Makes 4 servings
Prep Time: 5 minutes, plus soaking time
Total Time: 5 minutes

2 cups rolled oats
3 tablespoons chia seeds
½ teaspoon ground cinnamon
¼ cup golden raisins
¼ cup slivered almonds
1 Granny Smith apple, grated
2 ½ cups milk of choice
1 teaspoon vanilla extract
1 to 2 tablespoons raw honey

Place all the ingredients in a bowl and mix well to combine. Let the mixture sit overnight in the refrigerator before serving.

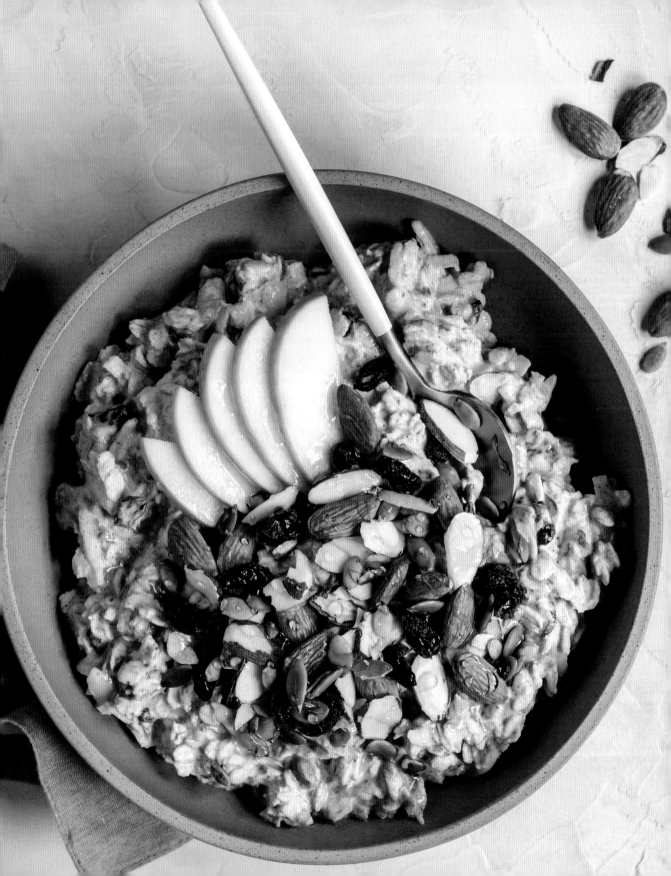

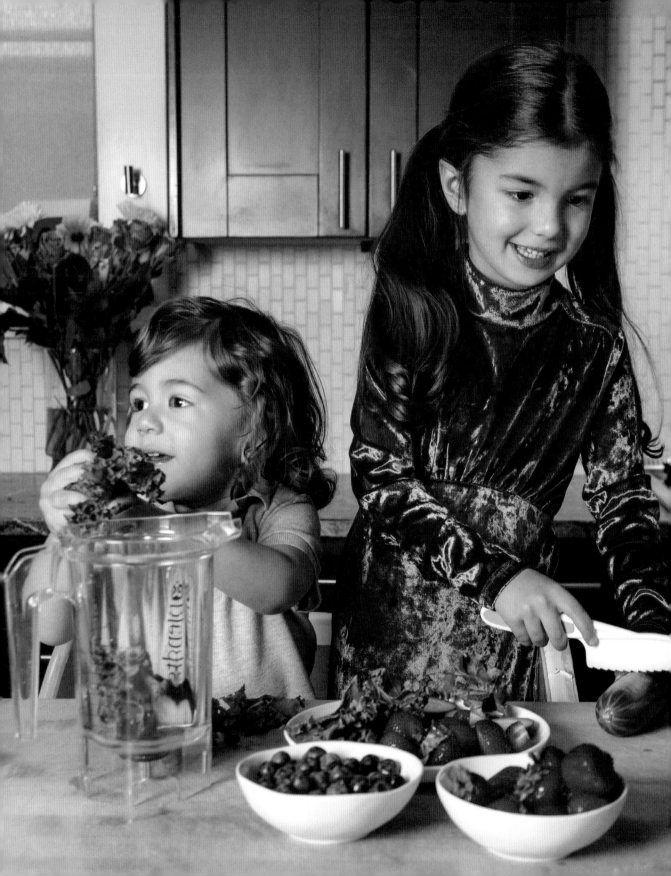

chapter 6

DRINKS, SMOOTHIES, AND MILKSHAKES

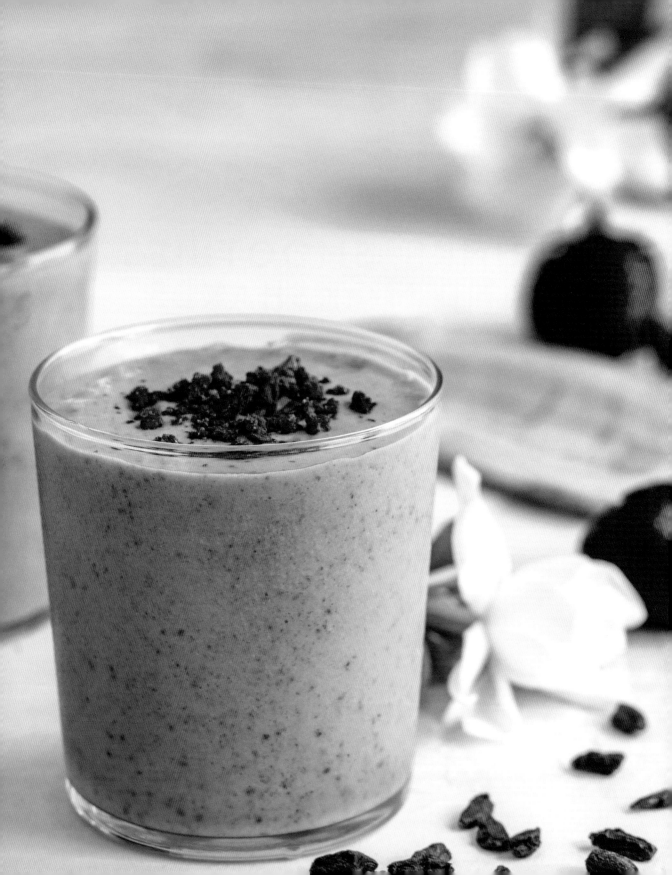

GOJI BERRY BLISS SMOOTHIE

Did you know that goji berries have one of the highest concentrations of antioxidants of any food? Antioxidants are very important because they fight all the free radicals and toxins you can accumulate in your body that cause aging and disease. Paired with organic strawberries, raw almond butter, and bananas, they make a delicious antioxidant-rich smoothie that will give you tons of energy.

Makes 1 serving
Prep Time: 5 minutes

1 cup frozen strawberries

1 ripe banana, peeled

2 tablespoons goji berries

1 tablespoon almond butter

½ cup coconut milk, more as needed

1 scoop Truvani protein powder and/ or 1 scoop Truvani marine collagen (optional)

Place all ingredients in a blender and blend until smooth.

SWEET TREAT JUICE

This is a perfect juice for the morning when you need a blast of energy and cleansing work. The beets go straight to the blood to help your body to fight off a myriad of ailments. This juice is deliciously sweet and refreshing, but feel free to throw in bitter greens like kale or parsley to cut down the sweetness.

Makes 2 servings
Prep Time: 10 minutes

2 beets, ends removed
4 celery stalks
1 cucumber, ends removed
1 apple, cored

Wash all veggies thoroughly.

Juice each ingredient in this order: beets, celery, cucumber, and apple. Stir the mixture before serving. Clean the juicer immediately.

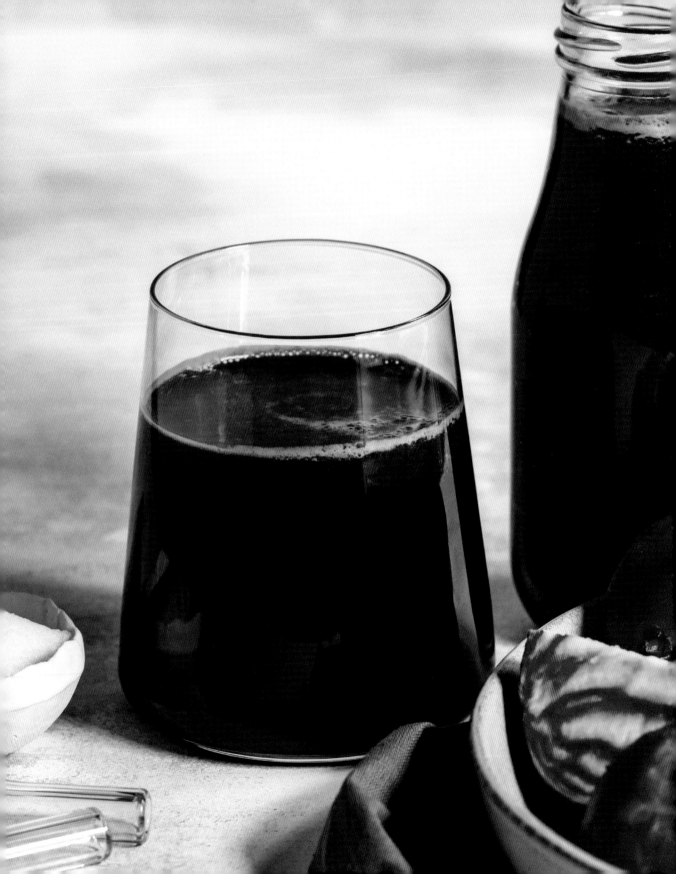

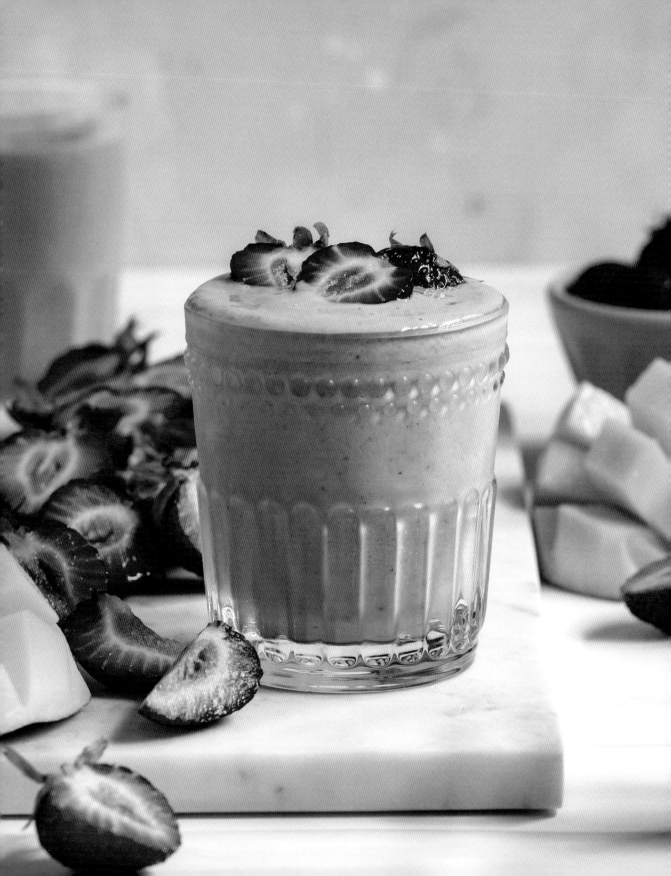

STRAWBERRY IMMUNE-BOOSTER SMOOTHIE

This smoothie is packed with immune system–boosting ingredients, such as strawberries, mango, and cauliflower, which are all high in vitamin C. And, trust me, putting cauliflower in a smoothie may sound weird, but it works beautifully! Plus, this smoothie includes probiotics from the yogurt, which help to improve gut health and keep your immune system strong!

Makes 2 servings
Prep Time: 5 minutes

1 cup frozen strawberries

1 ripe banana, peeled

½ cup frozen mango

½ cup frozen cauliflower florets

½ teaspoon ground turmeric

1 cup plain coconut yogurt

½ cup coconut milk, more as needed

1 scoop Truvani vanilla protein powder and/or Truvani marine collagen (optional)

Place all of the ingredients in a blender and blend until smooth.

CHOCOLATE PB SUPERFOOD SMOOTHIE

If you're having a hard time getting your child to try green drinks, this smoothie is a lifesaver! It tastes like a decadent chocolate milkshake, but it is packed with nutritious ingredients and greens. Want to save time? Skip the raw cacao and peanut butter and use Truvani Chocolate Peanut Butter Protein Powder instead.

Makes 2 servings
Prep Time: 5 minutes

2 frozen bananas, peeled

1 heaping cup of curly kale or baby spinach

3 tablespoons raw cacao powder

2 tablespoons peanut butter

2 tablespoons chia seeds

1 teaspoon vanilla extract

½ teaspoon ground cinnamon

½ cup nut milk or coconut milk, more as needed

Ice, as desired

1 scoop Truvani Chocolate Peanut Butter Protein Powder and/or Truvani marine collagen (optional)

Place all the ingredients in a blender and blend until smooth. Add ice if needed to reach desired consistency.

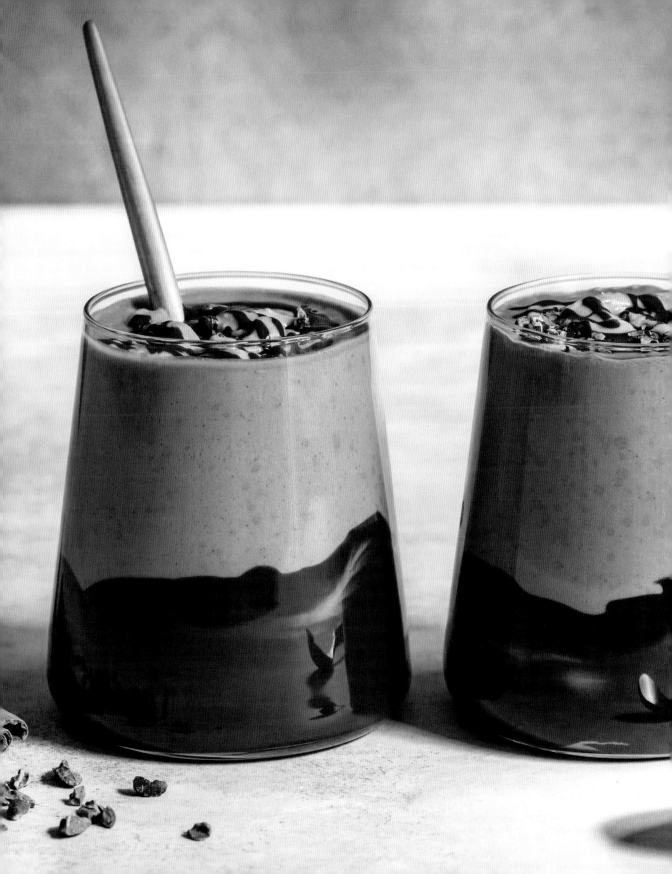

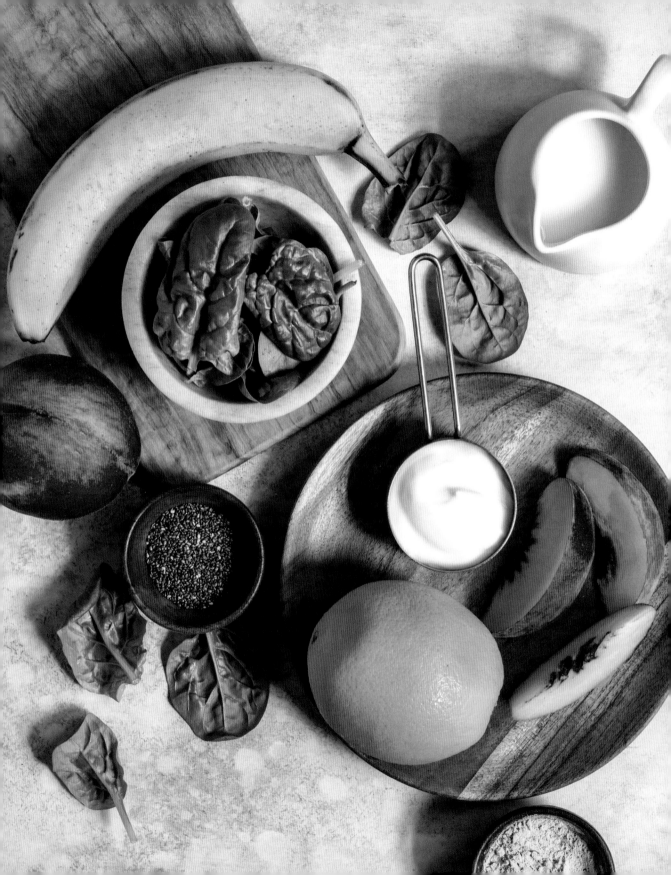

PEACHY GREEN SMOOTHIE

What a delicious way to get in your greens! Besides sneaking in a cup of spinach, this smoothie contains amazing chia seeds. These little seeds help you stay full for hours because they can grow 10 times their weight when combined with liquid. With their abundance of omega-3 fatty acids, chia seeds fight inflammation in the body, reducing the risk for many diseases.

Makes 1 serving
Prep Time: 5 minutes

1 peach, pitted
½ frozen banana, peeled
½ orange, peeled
1 cup spinach (or other leafy green)
1 tablespoon chia seeds
¼ cup plain yogurt of choice
¼ cup coconut milk, more as needed
1 scoop Truvani Protein + Greens or
1 scoop Truvani vanilla protein powder
(optional)

Place all the ingredients in a blender and blend until smooth.

BANANA BREAD SMOOTHIE

This smoothie is sweet and comforting, just like a slice of your favorite banana bread. It is super satisfying and will curb those cravings for highly sugary treats and junk food. It's a great one for kids who aren't sure about greens yet, since they should not be able to detect them at all!

Makes 1 serving
Prep Time: 5 minutes

1 frozen banana, peeled
1 cup baby spinach or curly kale
1 date, pitted
1 tablespoon ground flaxseeds
1 tablespoon almond butter
1 teaspoon vanilla extract
½ teaspoon ground cinnamon
Pinch of nutmeg
½ cup almond milk, more as needed
1 scoop Truvani vanilla protein powder and/or Truvani marine collagen (optional)

Place all of the ingredients in a blender and blend until smooth.

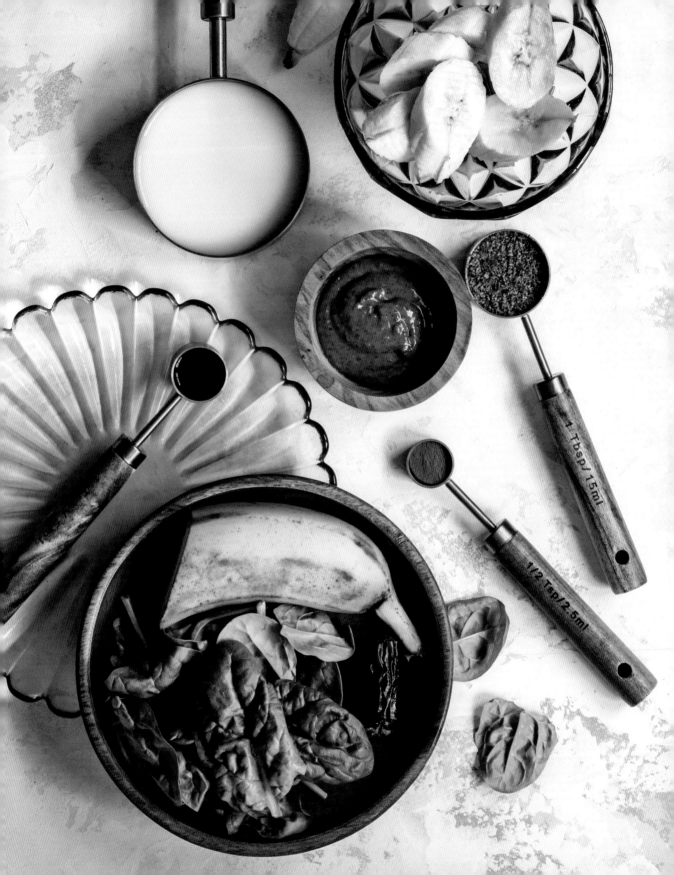

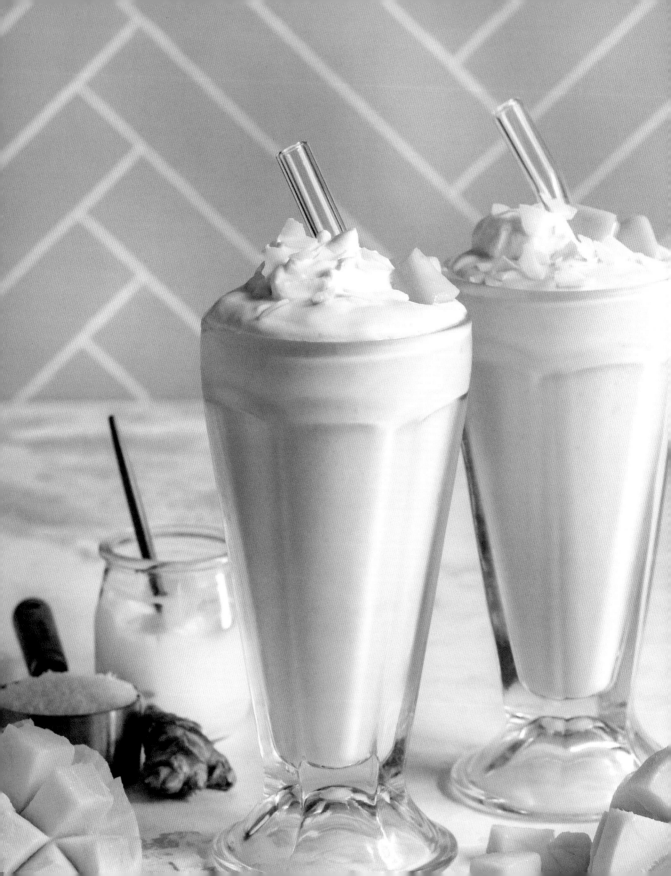

MANGO YOGURT MILKSHAKE

My mom used to make us a milkshake like this. It tastes like a frosty tropical dream, but is made with 100 percent healthy ingredients. The star ingredient here is the ginger root. I eat ginger almost every day: not only does it have a sweet and spicy taste that I love, but it's a master at fighting inflammation. A true superfood!

Makes 2 servings
Prep Time: 5 minutes

3 cups frozen chopped mango
1 cup plain yogurt of choice
1 teaspoon grated ginger root
¼ teaspoon ground cardamom
½ to ¾ cup coconut milk

Place all ingredients in a blender and blend until smooth.

HOMEMADE SPORTS DRINK

When I look at the ingredients in sports drinks, I just shake my head. Gatorade and Powerade are full of GMOs, artificial food dyes, and processed additives. No, thanks! This homemade sports drink is made with only fruits and vegetables, and it is perfect after a hot day in the sun or after a big game. It's naturally loaded with nutrients and electrolytes to replenish your body and get you hydrated fast, while giving you a serious dose of nutrition! (When I'm in a pinch, coconut water does the trick too for quick hydration.)

Makes 1 serving
Prep Time: 5 minutes

1 cup chopped seedless watermelon
1 apple, cored
½ cucumber
2 stalks celery
1 orange, peeled
2 cups chopped romaine lettuce

Wash all fruits and vegetables.

Place all ingredients through your juicer. Clean the juicer immediately.

You can prepare this ahead of time and keep chilled for up to 3 days.

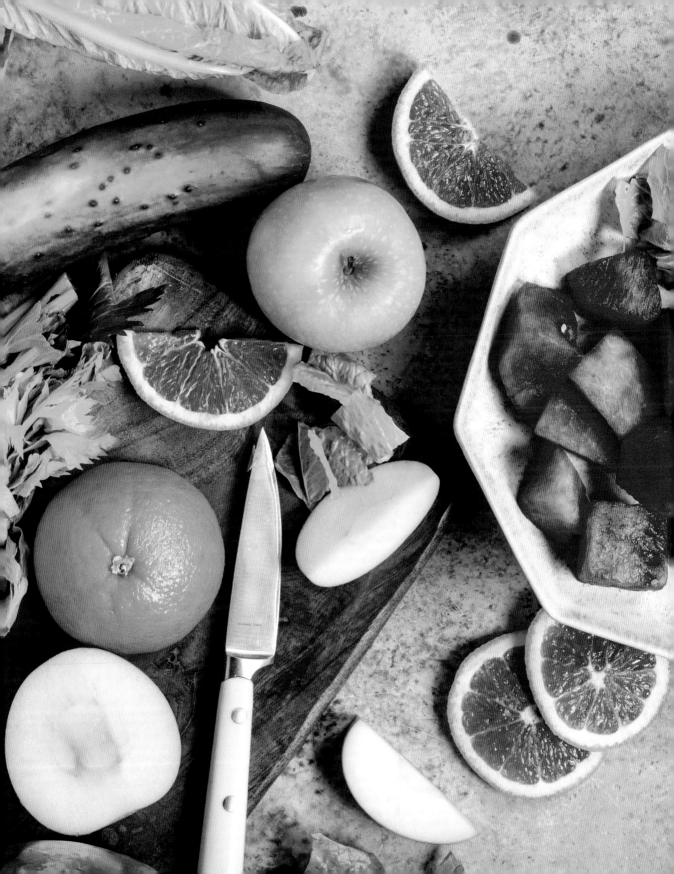

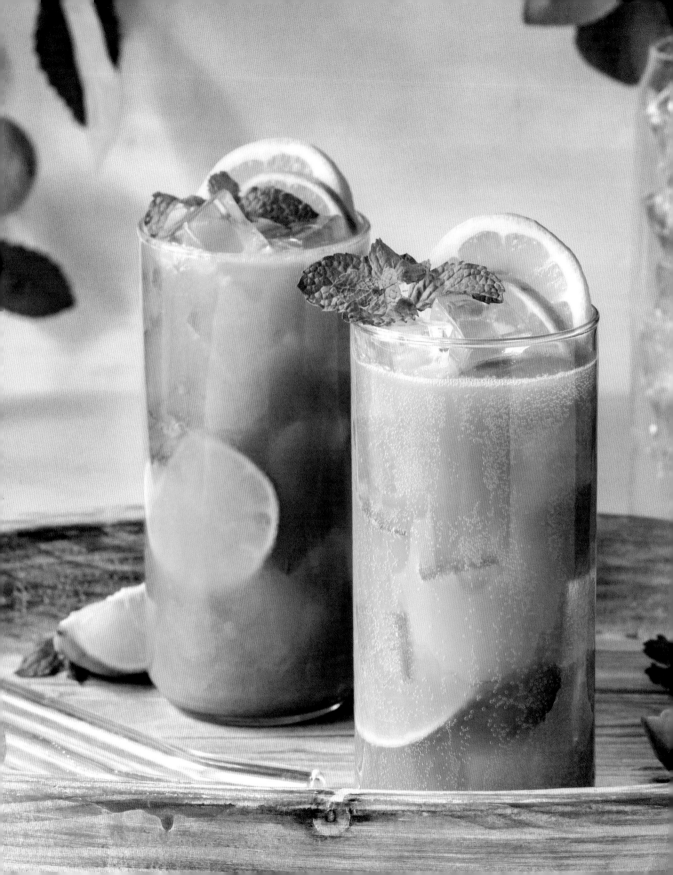

LEMON-LIME FIZZ

If you're addicted to sodas, this is a great way to enjoy the fizz without the nasty ingredients found in drinks like Sprite and 7UP. This recipe makes four servings, so you can make a batch of the lemon-lime mix and store it in your fridge for up to three days. When you're ready for a drink, simply whisk it into sparkling water and voilà! This one is great to serve at parties too.

Makes 4 servings
Prep Time: 5 minutes

1 small cucumber, ends trimmed and chopped
1 lemon, juiced
1 lime, juiced
1 green apple, peeled and cored
1 teaspoon raw honey (optional for additional sweetness)
16 ounces sparkling water
Mint leaves, for serving (optional)

Place all the ingredients except the sparkling water and mint leaves in a blender and blend until well combined. Strain through a fine mesh strainer. Taste and adjust with added honey, if needed.

Place some ice cubes in a glass and pour 4 ounces of the lemon-lime juice into the glass. Add 4 ounces of sparkling water and stir gently to combine. Top with a few mint leaves, if using.

FOOD BABE'S FAVORITE LUNCHTIME SMOOTHIE

This is the best smoothie for busy parents. I usually make this for myself and my husband because we are working from home. We usually drink this and then finish off whatever the kids are eating for lunch. This smoothie makes me feel absolutely amazing because it's chock-full of nutrients, anti-inflammatory ingredients, protein, collagen, and healthy fats—the perfect balanced lunch on busy days.

Makes 2 servings
Prep Time: 5 minutes

2 scoops Truvani Protein + Greens
2 scoops Truvani Marine Collagen
4 stalks celery, chopped
1 cucumber, chopped
1-inch piece ginger root
½ lemon, juiced
3 cups chopped kale, spinach, or greens of your choice
2 green apples, chopped and cored, or 2 cups mixed berries

Place all ingredients in a blender and blend until smooth.

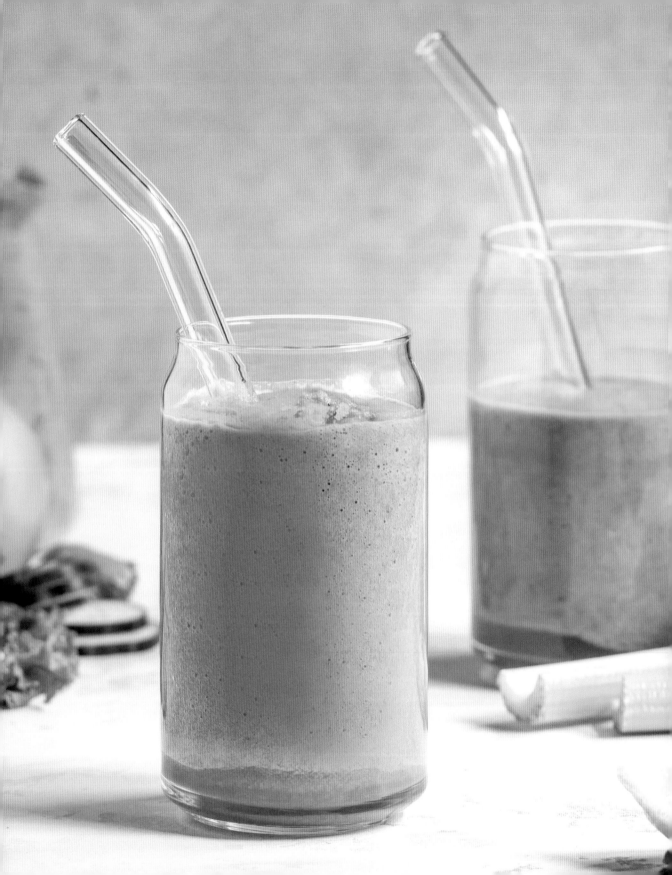

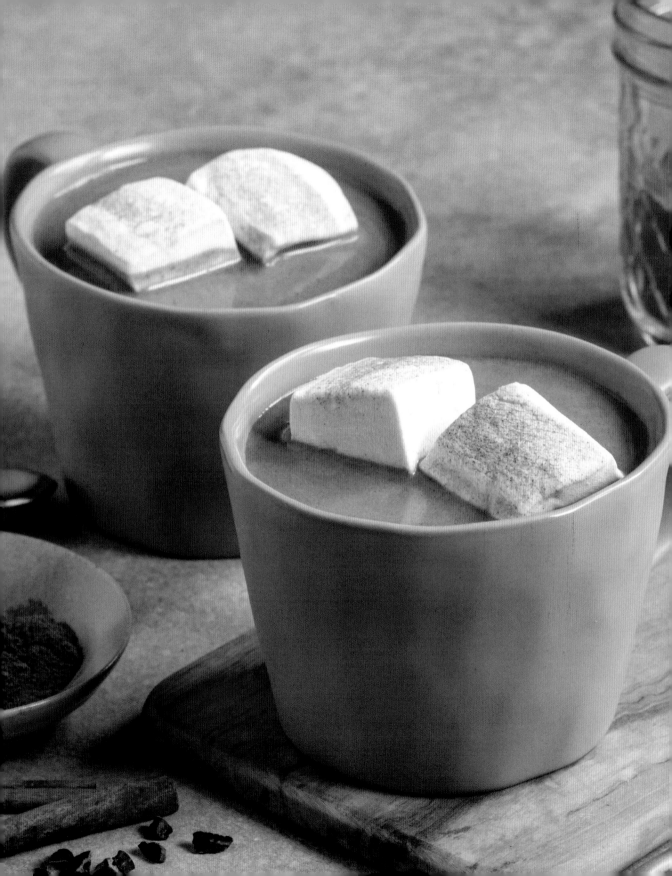

3-INGREDIENT HOT COCOA MIX

All the popular brands of hot cocoa mix are packed with unnecessary emulsifiers, refined sweeteners, and fake flavors. This is totally ridiculous! You can make hot cocoa with a handful of pantry ingredients—and this is how I make it at home nowadays. Stir up a big batch and store it in a glass jar for when the craving strikes!

Makes 18 servings
Prep Time: 5 minutes

1 cup cacao powder
1 cup coconut sugar
1 ½ cups coconut milk powder

Sift together the ingredients until well combined. Store in an airtight container or glass jar.

To make a cup of hot cocoa, heat 8 ounces of water and add 3 tablespoons of the cocoa mix. Stir well to combine.

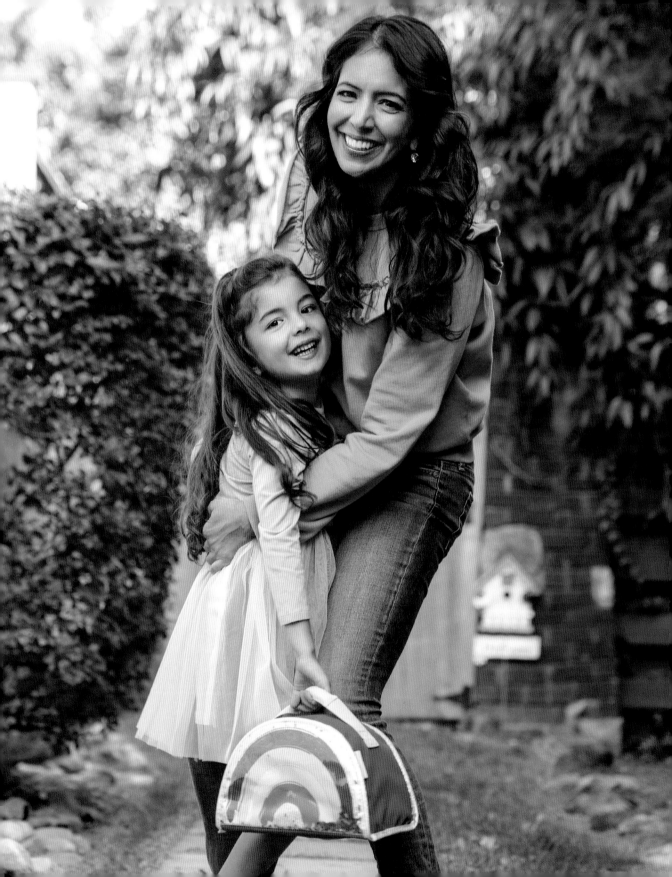

chapter 7

LUNCH BOXES

PINWHEELS (3 Ways)

Children love these pinwheels! Roll-ups are easy and fun to eat—a great option if your child doesn't have a long lunch break. I love to make them too, since they only take a handful of ingredients and a few minutes to assemble.

Here are three of my favorite fillings for roll-ups, which include healthy proteins and veggies to keep your child full and energetic for the rest of the school day. I would prep the ingredients ahead of time so they come together quickly on busy mornings.

HUMMUS, CUCUMBER, AND CARROT ROLL-UP

Makes 1 serving
Prep Time: 5 minutes

3 tablespoons hummus, divided
1 large sprouted-grain wrap (gluten-free: coconut or cassava wrap)
2 romaine lettuce leaves
1 carrot, shredded (¾ cup)
6 to 7 long, thin cucumber slices

Spread 2 tablespoons of hummus across the center of the wrap.

Top with the lettuce, shredded carrot, and sliced cucumber.

Spread 1 tablespoon of hummus across the top end of the wrap (this will help seal or "glue" the wrap once it is rolled).

Fold the bottom half of the wrap over the filling, tucking and rolling it tightly. Press down on the edge of the roll that has the hummus to seal the wrap. Cut the roll into 4 to 6 pinwheel slices.

SMASHED BLACK BEAN, CHEESE, AND AVOCADO ROLL-UP

Prep Time: 5 minutes

½ cup cooked black beans, roughly mashed
1 sprouted grain wrap (gluten-free: use coconut or cassava wrap)
2 romaine lettuce leaves
¾ cup grated goat cheddar cheese
1 small tomato, sliced
½ avocado, sliced
Sea salt and ground black pepper, to taste

Spread the mashed black beans across the center of the wrap.

Top with the lettuce, cheese, tomato, and avocado. Season with salt and pepper.

Fold the bottom half of the wrap over the filling, tucking and rolling tightly to enclose. Press roll to seal; cut into 4 to 6 pinwheel slices.

CHICKEN, BROCCOLI, AND ROASTED RED PEPPER ROLL-UP

Prep Time: 10 minutes
Cook Time: 12 to 15 minutes
Total Time: 22 to 25 minutes

1 cup chopped broccoli florets
½ red bell pepper, sliced
¼ red onion, sliced
1 to 2 tablespoons olive oil
Salt and pepper to taste
½ cup cooked diced chicken
1 sprouted-grain wrap (gluten-free: use coconut or cassava wrap)
2 tablespoons crumbled goat feta cheese

Preheat the oven to 400°F.

Place the broccoli, red pepper, and onion on a parchment-lined baking sheet. Drizzle with olive oil and toss to combine. Spread vegetables out in a single layer. Season with salt and pepper. Bake until the broccoli is golden brown and crispy, about 12 to 15 minutes.

Scatter chicken across the center of the wrap. Top with desired amount of the warm broccoli mix and the feta cheese.

Fold the bottom half of the wrap over the filling, tucking and rolling tightly to enclose. Press the roll to seal; cut into 4 to 6 pinwheel slices.

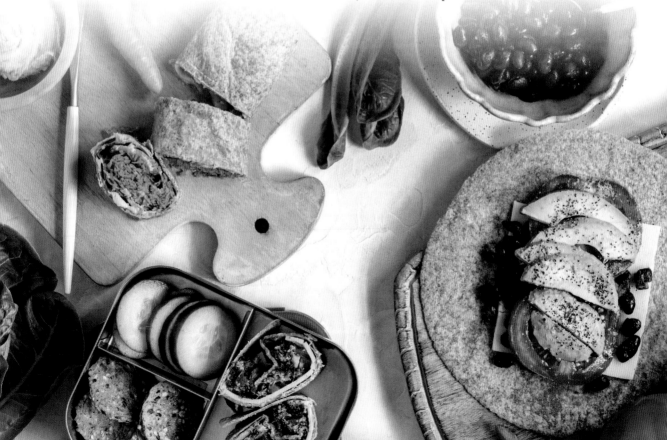

MEDITERRANEAN CHICKPEA SALAD

My daughter loves taking a little salad to school with her; the crunch of the cucumber and pine nuts is probably her favorite part. Feel free to leave out the pine nuts if your school is nut free. Pack this lunch with desired sides, such as a cheese stick, quinoa crackers, apple slices, or chocolate-covered nuts.

Makes 4 servings
Prep Time: 10 minutes

SALAD

1 ½ cups cooked chickpeas
1 small cucumber, diced
1 cup cherry tomatoes, halved
¼ cup kalamata olives, sliced (optional)
1 avocado, peeled, pitted, and diced
¼ cup pine nuts, toasted (optional)

Place all the salad ingredients in a bowl and toss to combine.

DRESSING

¼ cup extra virgin olive oil
2 tablespoons apple cider vinegar
1 tablespoon lemon juice
1 tablespoon chopped fresh parsley
½ teaspoon dried oregano
Sea salt and ground black pepper to taste

To make the dressing: Whisk together all the ingredients. Pour it over the salad and toss well.

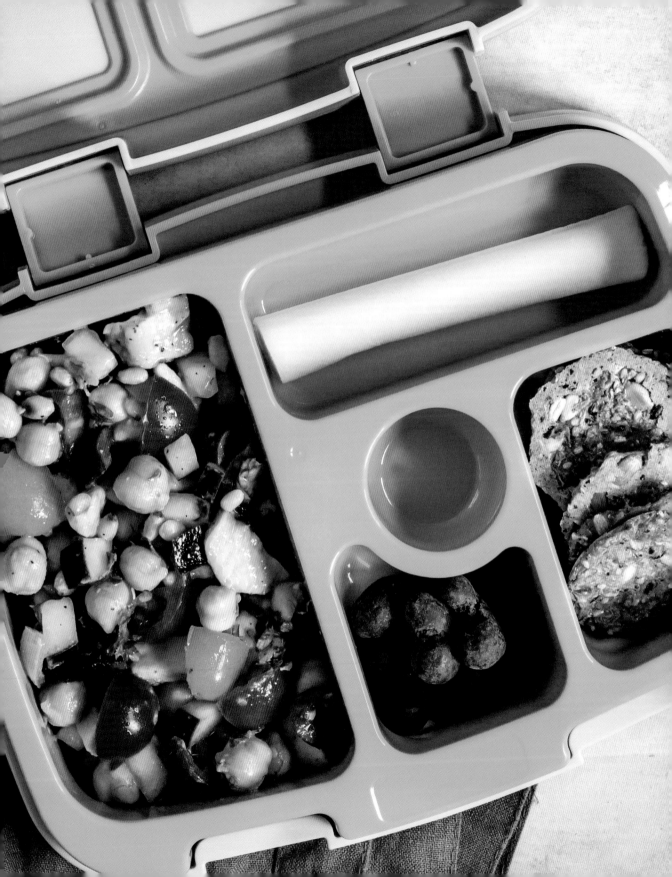

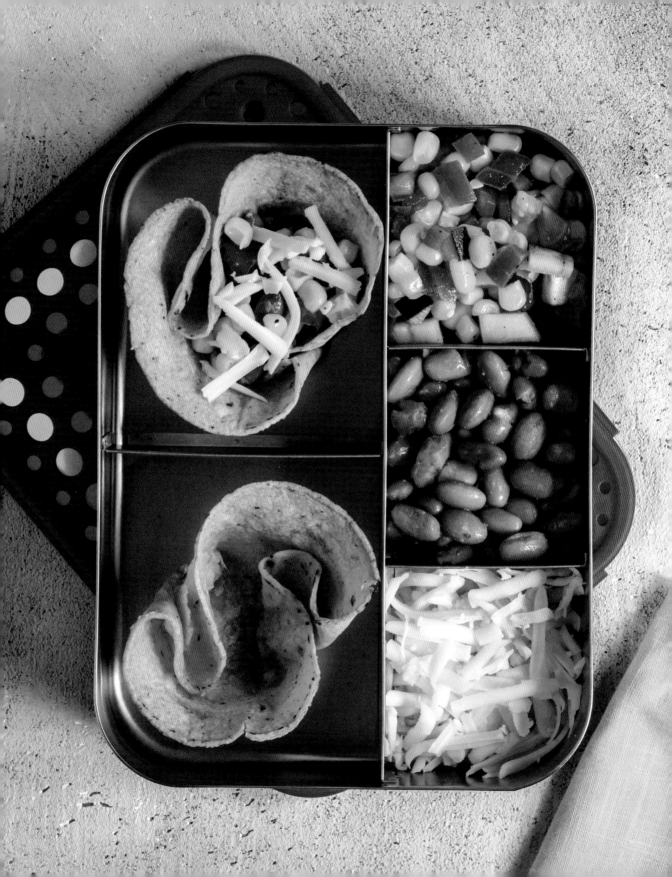

TACO SALAD CUPS

The beauty of this dish is that kids can have a little fun with it. I pack the taco cups, beans, corn salad, and cheese in separate compartments so Harley can have fun assembling the cups at school. Pack this lunch with sides, such as a piece of fresh fruit or beet chips.

Makes 4 servings
Prep Time: 20 minutes
Cook Time: 12 minutes
Total Time: 32 minutes

TORTILLA CUPS

8 sprouted corn tortillas
3 tablespoons olive oil

SALAD

1 cup sweet corn
1 small tomato, diced
½ small cucumber, diced
½ green bell pepper, diced
2 tablespoons chopped fresh basil
2 tablespoons extra-virgin olive oil
½ lime, juiced
Sea salt and freshly ground black pepper to taste
1 cup cooked beans of choice (such as black beans, pinto beans, cannellini beans)
¼ cup shredded goat cheddar cheese

Preheat the oven to 350°F.

Rub some olive oil into both sides of each tortilla to soften them and make them more pliable. In an unlined muffin tin, place each tortilla in a muffin cup, gently pushing down into the shape of the pan. Don't worry if the tortillas crack slightly; the shells should still hold together once baked. Bake until the edges are golden brown, about 10 to 12 minutes. Let the shells cool completely.

While the tortillas are baking, make the salad. Place the corn, tomato, cucumber, bell pepper, and basil in a bowl and mix to combine. Add the oil, lime juice, and a pinch of salt and pepper and toss well.

To assemble, take one of the crispy taco cups and add 2 tablespoons of the beans. Top with the veggie corn salad and ½ tablespoon of shredded cheese.

LENTIL PASTA
with Zucchini and Tomato Sauce

This is the easiest main lunch dish I make for my children, with two items I always have stocked in my pantry. If the week's groceries are going right, I'll try to get some extra vegetables into the sauce. I can't say I do that every time—but the weeks I do, I feel like a superstar.

Makes 2 servings
Prep Time: 5 minutes
Cook Time: 10 minutes
Total Time: 15 minutes

4 ounces lentil pasta

1 medium zucchini, ends trimmed and chopped

1 cup Lucini tomato sauce

Cook the pasta according to the directions on the package.

In a small pot, steam the zucchini until it's tender. Drain and place the cooked zucchini in a blender and puree it.

Add the zucchini and sauce to the pasta and heat until warmed through.

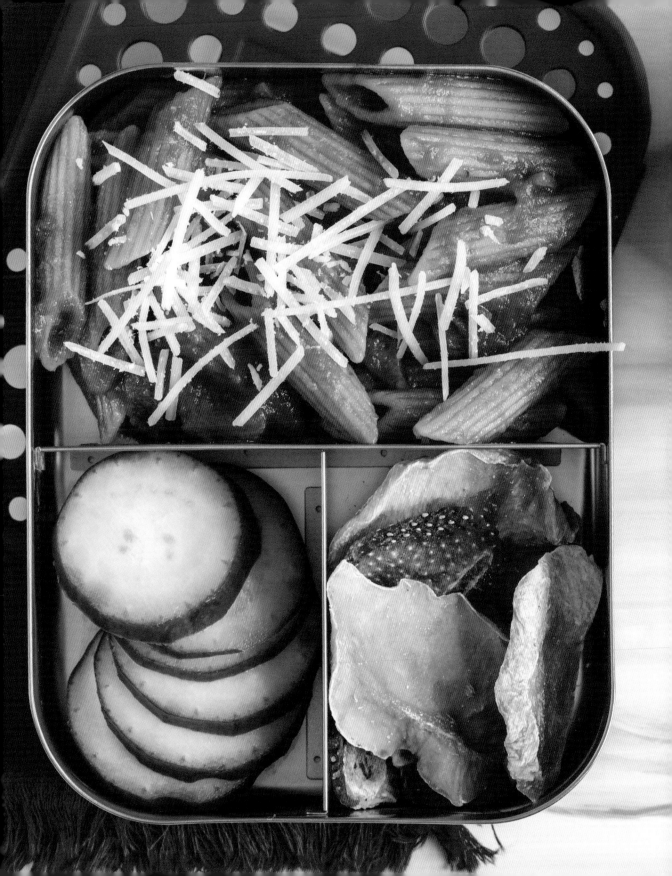

PINTOS AND RICE IN A THERMOS

This is a nice hot lunch option that I can make with a staple that can be found in my freezer. I freeze individual portions of the Pinto Beans (page 259) to have available at all times. Pair with your rice of choice and/or the sautéed veggies in the Veggie Fajitas recipe (page 239).

Makes 1 serving
Prep Time: 5 minutes

½ cup pinto beans (recipe on page 259)
½ cup cooked rice
½ to 1 cup sautéed vegetables (optional)
1 to 2 tablespoons of shredded cheddar cheese

Place the beans, rice, and vegetables in a thermos and mix to combine.

Pack this lunch with the shredded cheese on the side so that your child can have fun sprinkling it on top.

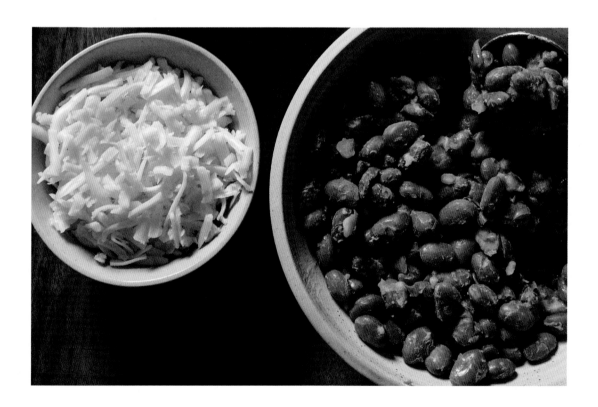

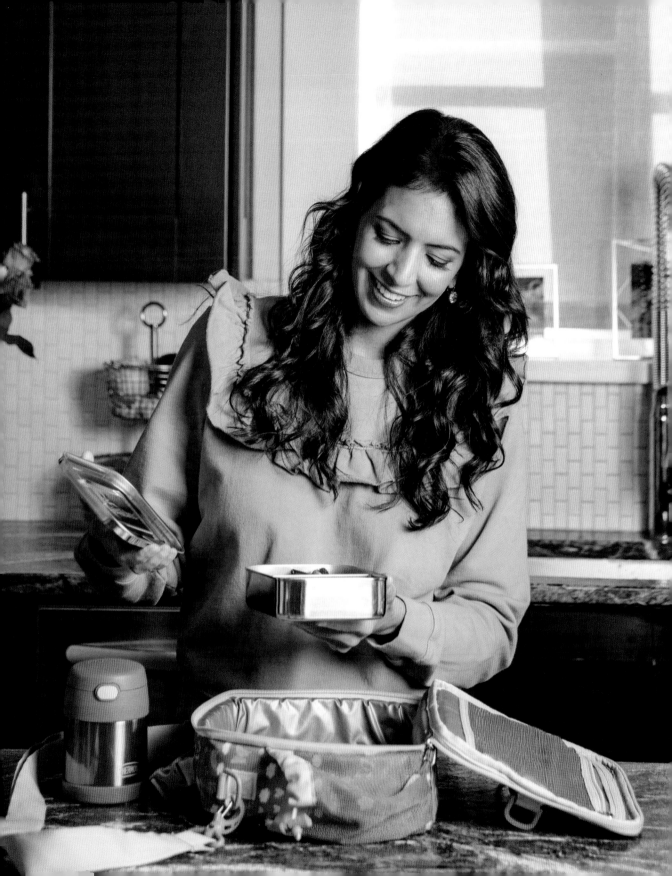

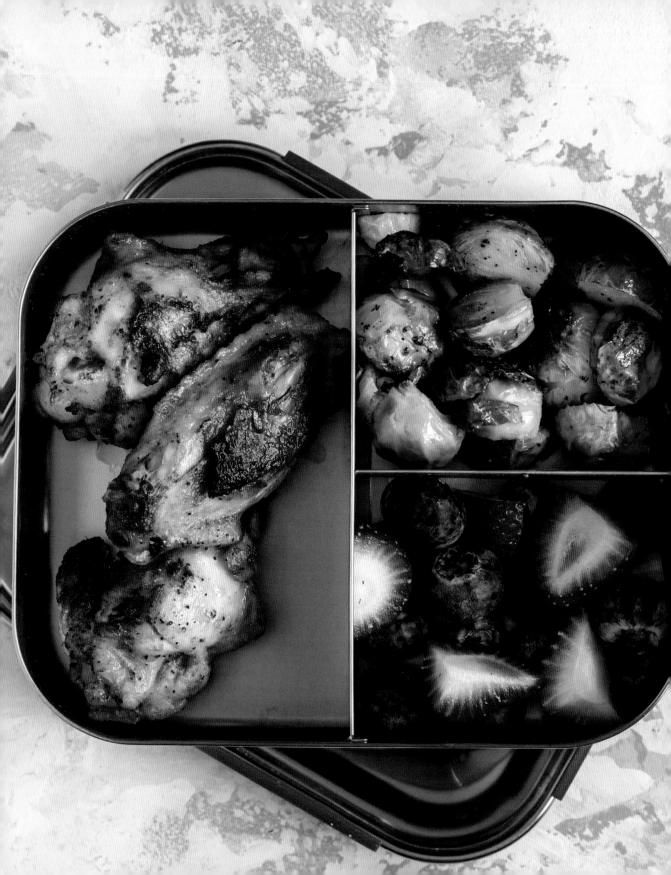

CHICKEN WINGS
with Roasted Brussels Sprouts

Everyone in my house goes gaga over chicken wings. Even when served cold they still taste good. But I usually roast the brussels sprouts in the morning and toss them a thermos to keep them warm for lunch at school.

Makes 4 to 6 servings
Prep Time: 75 minutes
Cook Time: 30 minutes
Total Time: 1 hour 45 minutes

2 tablespoons olive oil
1 teaspoon sea salt
½ teaspoon paprika
Ground black pepper to taste
1 lemon, juiced
2 pounds chicken wings

Preheat the oven to 425°F.

In a bowl, combine the olive oil, seasonings, and lemon juice. Let the wings marinate in the refrigerator for at least 1 hour.

Place the wings in a baking pan or on a parchment-lined baking sheet and bake them for 15 minutes per side.

ROASTED BRUSSELS SPROUTS

16 ounces brussels sprouts, ends trimmed and cut in half
1 bulb garlic, broken into cloves and peeled
1 to 2 tablespoons olive oil
Sea salt and ground black pepper to taste

Place the brussels sprouts and garlic cloves on a parchment-lined baking sheet and toss with the oil, salt, and pepper. Bake them in the oven with the wings for 15 minutes.

SALMON BALLS

I worried so much that Harley's lunch would be the "stinky fish" one at school, but thankfully, these aren't as odoriffic as I thought they would be. This has turned out to be one of Harley's favorite school lunches, and it is so fun for her to eat. You can use Japanese onigiri molds in the shape of triangles, hearts, flowers, or squares for a different take on the "ball" shape.

Makes 4 to 6 servings
Prep Time: 15 minutes
Cook Time: 30 minutes
Total Time: 45 minutes

1 cup Lundberg sushi rice
16 ounces Patagonia wild-caught cooked salmon, chopped (you can also use leftover cooked wild-caught salmon)

Make the rice according to the directions on the package. Skip using butter when making the rice. Let it cool to room temperature.

Take a handful of rice, roughly ¼ cup, and form a ball. Make a small indent in the center of the ball for the salmon. Place roughly 1 to 2 tablespoons of the chopped salmon in the indent. Cover the indent with some more rice and squeeze it all together to form a ball again. You can use a small bowl of water to wet your hands so the rice doesn't stick to them. Repeat until you have used the remaining ingredients.

If you are using nigiri molds, take some of the rice and fill the mold halfway full, pressing down firmly into the mold. Add 1 to 2 tablespoons of the chopped salmon. Place more rice on top, pressing down until the mold is filled to the top.

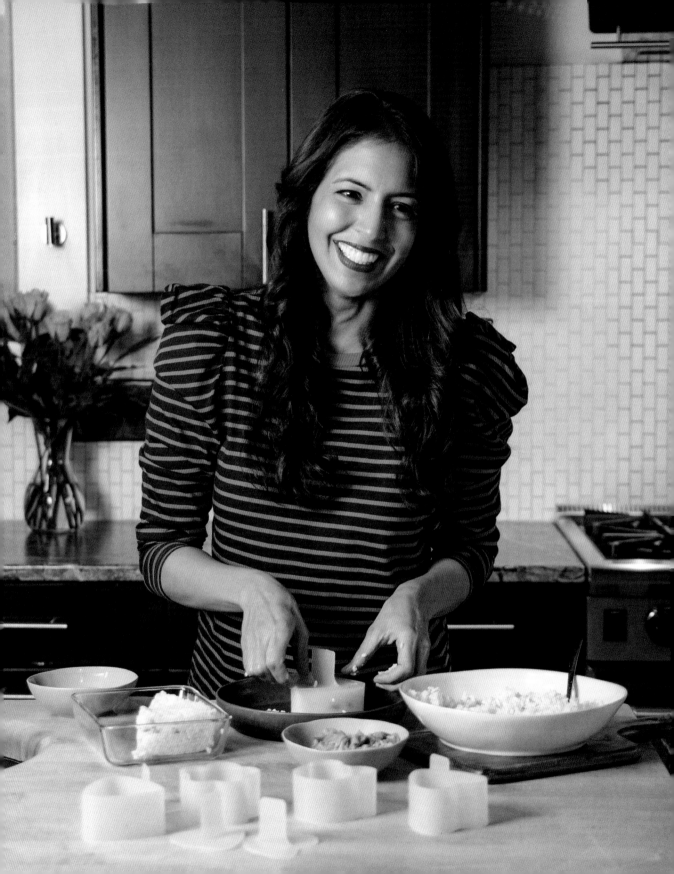

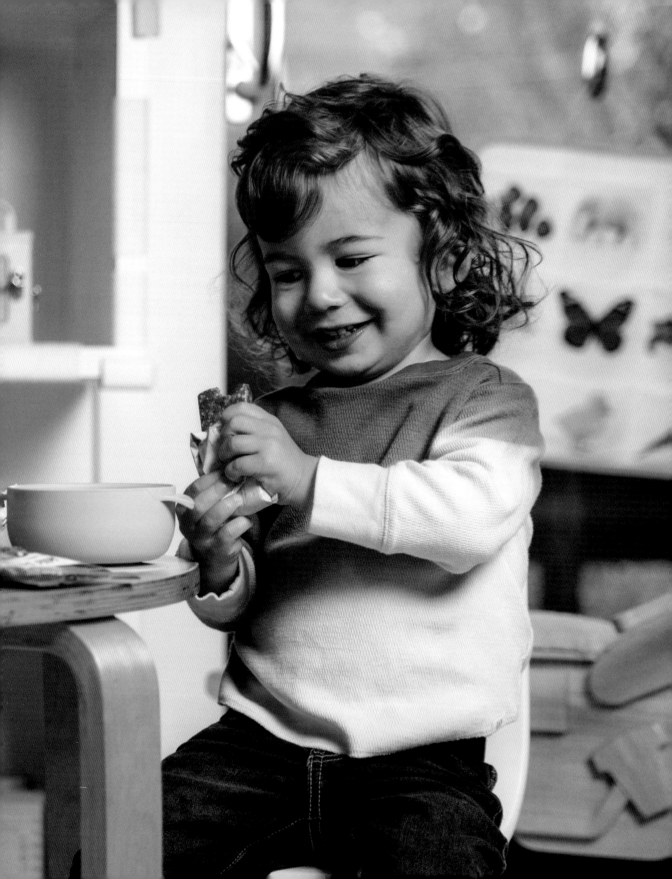

chapter 8

KID SNACKS

CRISPY RANCH CHICKPEAS

This crunchy, crispy, flavorful snack is a million times better than a bag of chips full of MSG, fake flavors, and dyes. It's a great source of protein and fiber too. Tasty *and* healthy is a win-win! My two-year-old loves to snack on these.

Makes 4 to 6 servings
Prep Time: 5 minutes
Cook Time: 30 minutes
Total Time: 35 minutes

CHICKPEAS

2 cups cooked chickpeas
2 tablespoons olive oil
2 tablespoons Homemade Ranch Seasoning, more as desired

HOMEMADE RANCH SEASONING

2 tablespoons buttermilk powder
1 tablespoon dried parsley
½ tablespoon onion powder
1 teaspoon garlic powder
1 teaspoon dried chives
½ teaspoon dried dill
½ teaspoon sea salt
¼ teaspoon ground black pepper

Preheat the oven to 425°F.

In a small bowl, mix together all the ingredients for the Homemade Ranch Seasoning. Set aside.

If using canned chickpeas, drain the liquid; then rinse and dry the chickpeas well. Place the chickpeas in a bowl and drizzle them with the olive oil. Sprinkle the ranch seasoning on top and toss to combine. Place on a parchment-lined baking sheet.

Bake for 25 to 30 minutes or until the chickpeas are golden brown and crispy. Serve immediately. After they cool fully, you can store them in an airtight container for up to 2 days.

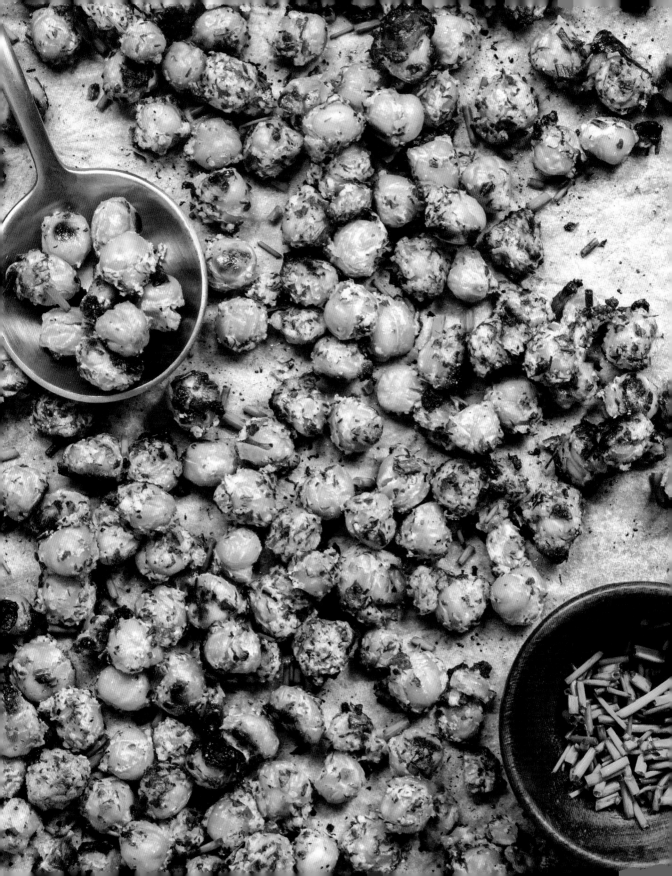

HOMEMADE PEANUT BUTTER & JAM

Sometimes there is nothing more comforting than this throwback to my elementary school days: the classic peanut-butter sandwich. Nowadays, though, I don't use Peter Pan peanut butter spiked with hydrogenated oils or Smucker's jam sweetened with high-fructose corn syrup. Yuck! Who knew it was so easy to make my own peanut butter and jam?

Makes 4 to 6 servings
Prep Time: 10 to 20 minutes
Cook Time: 15 minutes
Total Time: 25 to 40 minutes

3 cups dry-roasted peanuts
Sea salt to taste

To make the peanut butter: Place the peanuts and salt in a food processor and process on high until smooth and creamy (about 10 to 20 minutes), scraping the sides every minute.

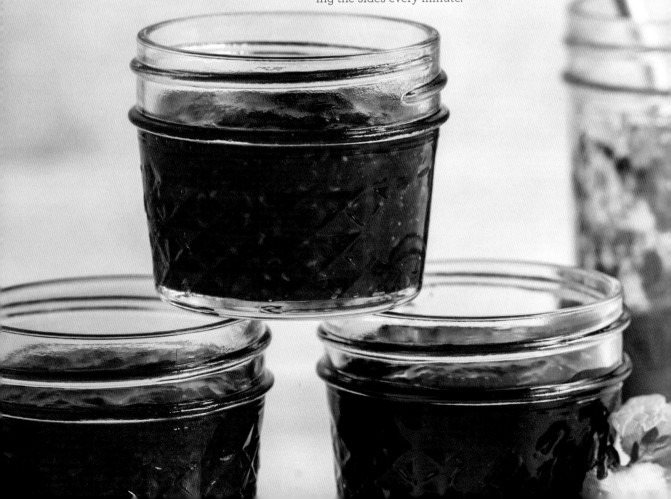

STRAWBERRY JAM

3 cups halved strawberries
2 tablespoons lemon juice
2 tablespoons raw honey

BLUEBERRY JAM

2 ½ cups blueberries
2 tablespoons lemon juice
2 tablespoons raw honey

RASPBERRY JAM

1 ½ cups raspberries
2 tablespoons lemon juice
2 tablespoons raw honey

MIXED BERRY JAM

3 cups mixed berries
2 tablespoons lemon juice
2 tablespoons raw honey

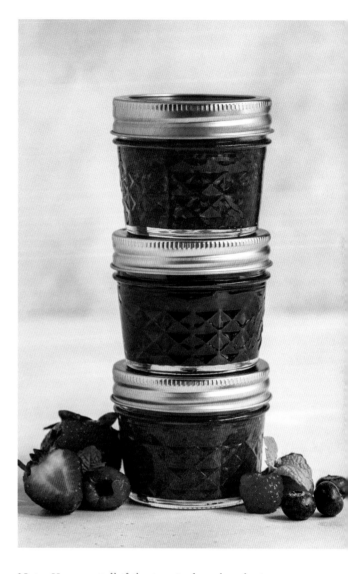

To make your jam of choice: Place all the ingredients in a small pot over medium heat. Cook until the fruit begins to break down, mashing it slightly to release the juices. Turn the heat to low and continue to cook for 15 to 20 minutes or until it has thickened.

Note: You can tell if the jam is done by placing the back of a clean spoon in the jam and making a path down the center of it with the spoon. If the path remains clean that means it's thick enough. Frozen fruit will take longer. Take the pot off the heat and let it cool. Store in a glass jar in the refrigerator for up to 1 week.

ZUCCHINI PIZZA BITES

Zap away any pizza craving with these little bites that are not only tasty but FUN to eat. Prepare a batch to share while watching a movie or playing a game with your family. These also make a great healthy alternative to processed "pizza rolls," which are full of sketchy ingredients.

Makes 4 to 6 servings
Prep Time: 5 minutes
Cook Time 20 minutes
Total Time: 25 minutes

1 zucchini, cut into ¼-inch-thick rounds
½ cup thick pizza sauce
4 ounces goat mozzarella cheese, cubed
¼ cup grated Parmesan cheese
Italian seasoning for topping

Preheat the oven to 400°F.

Arrange the zucchini rounds on a parchment-lined baking sheet. Top each with ½ tablespoon of pizza sauce and 1 mozzarella cube. Sprinkle the Parmesan and a pinch of Italian seasoning on top.

Bake for 18 to 22 minutes or until the cheese has melted and the zucchini is fork tender.

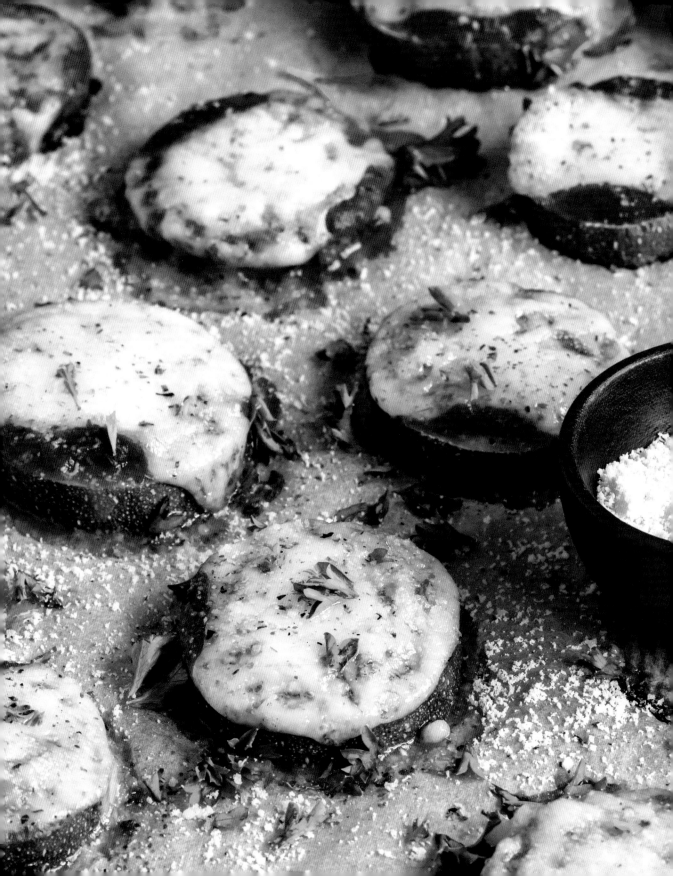

HEALTHY 7-LAYER DIP

This dip is absolutely fabulous for a get-together or BBQ—it's fun to prepare and gives you a good opportunity to indulge in a load of vegetables when the party's just getting started! I snuck in a layer of kale . . . I promise no one will notice. I like serving this with organic corn chips and celery sticks. I alternate between the two so I don't eat too many chips in one sitting!

Makes 12 to 15 servings
Prep Time: 20 minutes

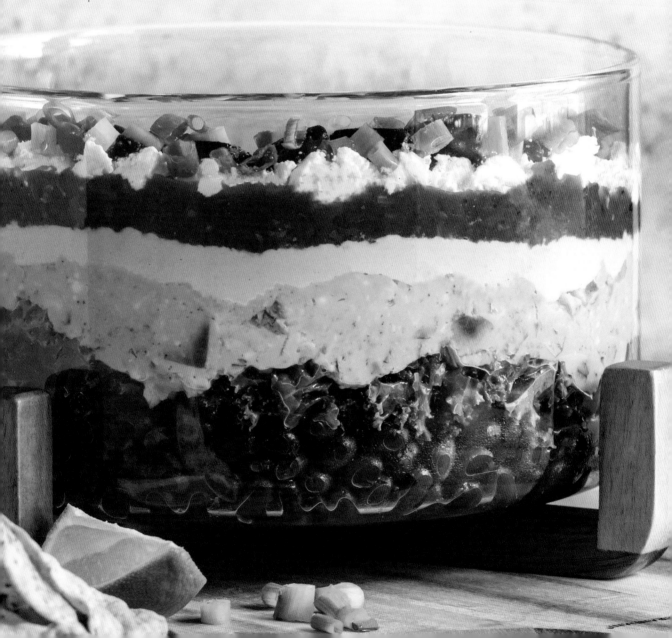

3 cups cooked black beans

2 teaspoons ground cumin

1 teaspoon chili powder

Sea salt and ground black pepper, to taste

1 cup finely chopped kale

2 cups finely chopped romaine lettuce

2 tablespoons extra virgin olive oil

1 clove garlic, minced

4 avocados, peeled and pitted

1 tomato, diced

½ cup diced red onion

1 lime, juiced

¼ cup chopped cilantro

16 ounces plain hummus

32 ounces salsa, drained

1 cup crumbled goat feta cheese

½ cup chopped Kalamata olives

¼ cup chopped scallions

Place the black beans in a bowl and add the cumin, chili powder, and a few shakes of salt and pepper. With a masher or the back of a spoon slightly mash the black beans. Set aside.

In a separate bowl, combine the kale, romaine, oil, and garlic, and massage the kale mix until it starts to soften. Set aside.

In another bowl, mash the avocado with the back of a spoon. Add the tomato, onion, lime juice, and cilantro. Mix and season with salt and pepper to taste. Set aside.

To assemble the dip, take a medium glass bowl (try to find one with straight sides) and spread the black beans on the bottom. Top that with the kale mix and then the avocado mix. Next, carefully spread the hummus on top, followed by the salsa. Sprinkle the goat cheese, olives, and scallions over the salsa. Serve with tortilla chips, crackers, or veggie sticks.

SUPERFOOD POPCORN

Making your own popcorn from scratch is so easy, and you can avoid the health pitfalls found in most bagged and microwave versions—dreadful oils and risky preservatives. If you need to take some to the office or wherever you are going (like sneaking it into the movie theater!), I recommend preparing it at home and throwing it into a reusable bag.

Makes 4 servings
Prep Time: 5 minutes
Cook Time: 5 minutes
Total Time: 10 minutes

1 tablespoon coconut oil
½ cup dry popcorn kernels
1 tablespoon hemp seeds
¼ teaspoon sea salt
1 tablespoon grass-fed butter

In a pot, stir together the coconut oil and popcorn kernels. and heat over medium-high heat.

Cover the pot with a lid and let the popcorn pop until you hear less popping per second. Remove the pot from the stove and pour the popcorn into a bowl.

Using a blender or food processor, blend the hemp seeds and salt until you get a fine powder. Top the popcorn with melted butter and dust it with the hemp seed mixture.

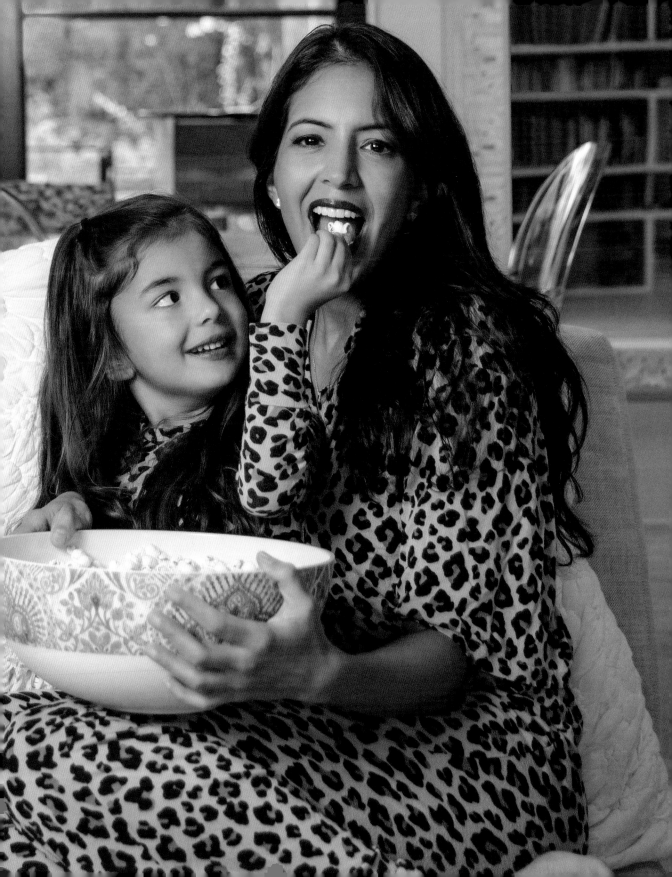

SLOW COOKER SOUTHWEST BLACK BEAN DIP

This bean dip is virtually effortless to make. You basically throw the ingredients in a small slow cooker, and when you come back in a couple hours it's practically ready to go. Serve this with raw veggie sticks and organic corn chips. You're going to love having this recipe in your back pocket when you need an easy appetizer or side, especially considering that most bean dips at the store are full of processed ingredients and artificial dyes. And if you don't have a slow cooker, don't worry—I've got you covered!

Makes 4 servings
Prep Time: 15 minutes
Cook Time: 2 hours
Total Time: 2 hours 15 minutes

1 ½ cups cooked black beans

1 cup of shredded goat cheddar cheese or grass-fed cheese

1 tomato, peeled, seeded, and diced

½ yellow onion, diced

¼ cup chopped scallions

¼ cup chopped fresh cilantro

2 cloves garlic, minced

1 teaspoon ground cumin

½ teaspoon sea salt

¼ teaspoon cayenne pepper

¼ teaspoon ground black pepper

Optional Toppings

1 tablespoon fresh lime juice

Hot sauce, to taste

2 tablespoons chopped fresh cilantro

1 tablespoon chopped scallions

2 tablespoons pumpkin seeds (pepitas)

Place all the ingredients in the slow cooker and cook on high for 2 hours or until the cheese is melted. (If you don't have a slow cooker, the ingredients can be mixed in a 6-cup ceramic or glass baking dish, then covered and baked at 300°F until the veggies are very soft, about 1 hour.)

Using a potato masher, mash the bean mixture and transfer it to a bowl. Serve it plain or mix the lime juice and/or hot sauce into the dip. Garnish the dip with cilantro, scallions, and/or pumpkin seeds (all are optional). Serve with tortilla chips or raw veggies.

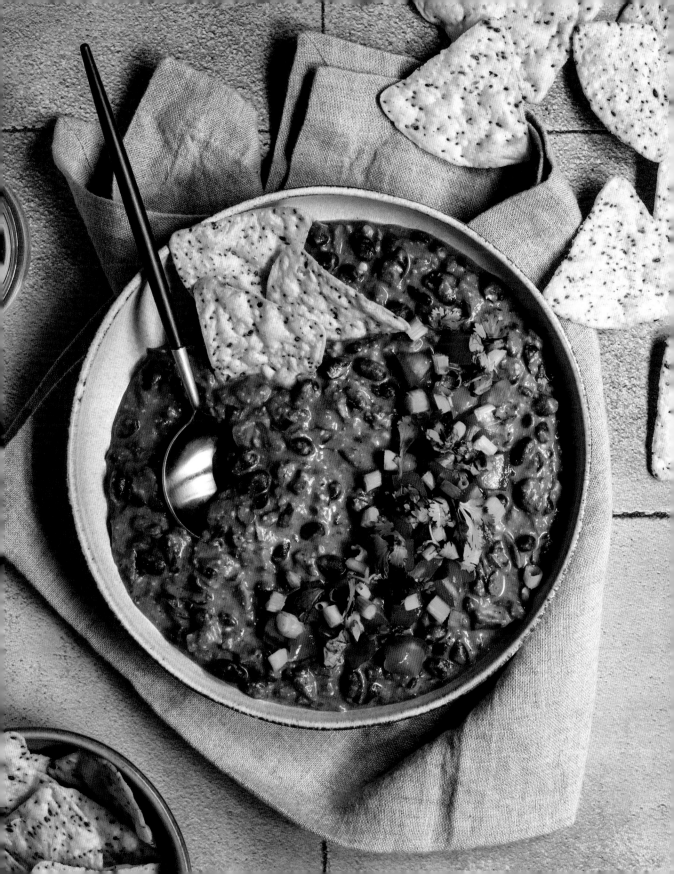

VEGGIES WITH 5 EFFORTLESS DIPS

Dips are a must-have for children (and us parents too!). It's so much more fun to eat veggies when you've got a tasty dip to dig into. Get creative with the veggies you serve; you don't need to stick with carrots and celery all the time. Try radishes, bell peppers, cucumbers, cauliflower, snap peas, jicama, and zucchini. These dips also go great with sprouted-grain pita chips and rice crackers.

Makes 1 to 2 cups dip
Prep Time: 10 minutes

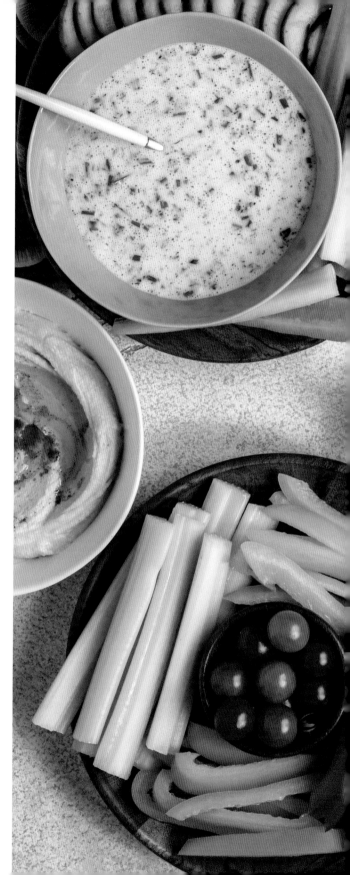

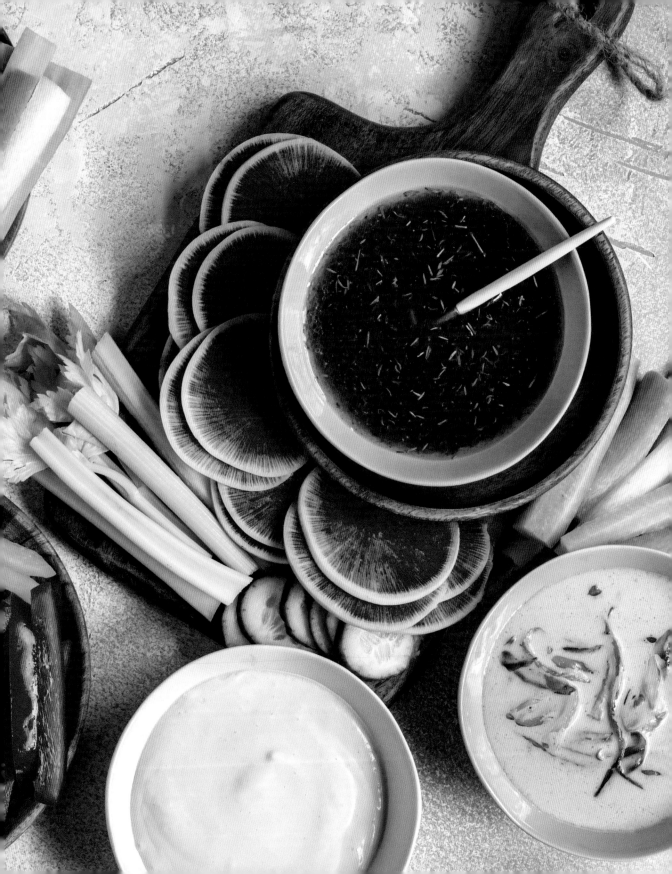

RANCH DIP

¼ cup buttermilk powder
1 tablespoon dried parsley
½ tablespoon onion powder
1 teaspoon garlic powder
1 teaspoon dried chives
½ teaspoon dried dill
½ teaspoon sea salt
¼ teaspoon ground black pepper
1 cup mayo (look for one made with avocado oil)
1 cup milk

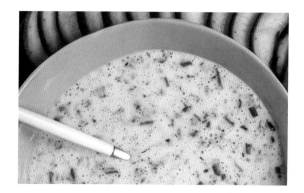

Place all the dry ingredients in a bowl and mix well.

In a separate bowl, add the mayo and milk and mix well. Add 2½ tablespoons of the spice mix to the wet ingredients and whisk to combine. Serve with veggie sticks or desired accompaniment.

SOUR CREAM & ONION DIP

1 to 2 tablespoons olive oil
1 large yellow onion, sliced thin
2 garlic cloves, minced
¼ teaspoon sea salt
½ teaspoon dried thyme
1 tablespoon balsamic vinegar
1 tablespoon coconut aminos
1 cup plain Greek yogurt

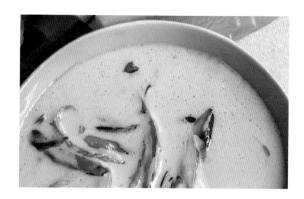

Heat the oil in a sauté pan over medium heat. Add the onions and let them cook for 4 to 5 minutes.

Add the remaining ingredients except the yogurt. Turn the heat to low and cook for 12 to 15 minutes or until the onions have caramelized. Let the mixture cool.

In a bowl, add the yogurt. Once the onions have cooled, add them to the bowl and mix well. Serve with veggie sticks or desired accompaniment.

EASY HOMEMADE HUMMUS

1½ cups cooked garbanzo beans
¼ cup tahini
1 garlic clove, minced
1 lemon, juiced
2 tablespoons extra virgin olive oil
¼ teaspoon sea salt
Pinch of ground black pepper

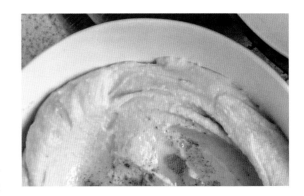

Place all the ingredients in a blender or food processor and blend until smooth and creamy. Serve with veggie sticks or desired accompaniment.

AVOCADO DIP

2 avocados, peeled and pitted
½ cup plain Greek yogurt
1 garlic clove, peeled
½ lime, juiced
¼ teaspoon sea salt

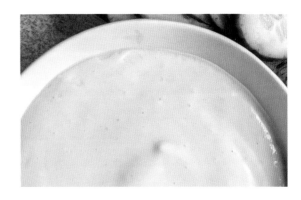

Place all the ingredients in a blender or food processor and blend until smooth and creamy. Serve with veggie sticks or desired accompaniment.

BALSAMIC VINEGAR DIP

½ cup extra virgin olive oil
5 tablespoons balsamic vinegar
1 tablespoon Dijon mustard
¼ teaspoon ground thyme
Sea salt and ground black pepper, to taste

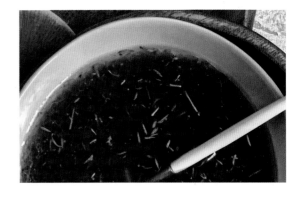

Place all of the ingredients in a small bowl and whisk together until fully combined. Serve with veggie sticks or desired accompaniment.

CHEESY CRACKERS
(aka Homemade Goldfish)

I developed this recipe because practically every child in the United States eats store-bought Gold-fish crackers made with ridiculously processed ingredients. I personally don't ever want to buy those for my kids, and so many of you feel the same and have asked for an alternative. I use a 1-inch-wide fish-shaped cookie cutter to make these. You could certainly use any cookie cutter shape you want for more variety and fun.

Makes 8 to 10 servings
Prep Time: 45 minutes
Cook Time: 15 minutes
Total Time: 60 minutes

1 cup spelt flour
6 tablespoons cold unsalted butter, cut into small pieces
8 ounces sharp cheddar cheese
¼ teaspoon onion powder
¼ teaspoon garlic powder
¼ teaspoon paprika
½ teaspoon sea salt
¼ teaspoon ground black pepper
3 to 4 tablespoons cold, filtered water

Preheat the oven to 350°F.

Place all the ingredients in a bowl. Using a pastry cutter, mix together the ingredients until the dough resembles a coarse meal. Alternatively, you can use a food processor if desired.

Add 3 to 4 tablespoons of cold water, one at a time, and mix until the dough forms a ball. Chill the dough in the refrigerator for at least 30 minutes.

Roll out the dough on a floured surface until it is roughly ⅛ inch thick. Use a cookie cutter to cut shapes out of the dough.

Place the shapes on a parchment-lined baking sheet and bake them for 15 to 18 minutes or until they are golden brown. Store in an airtight container for up to 2 days.

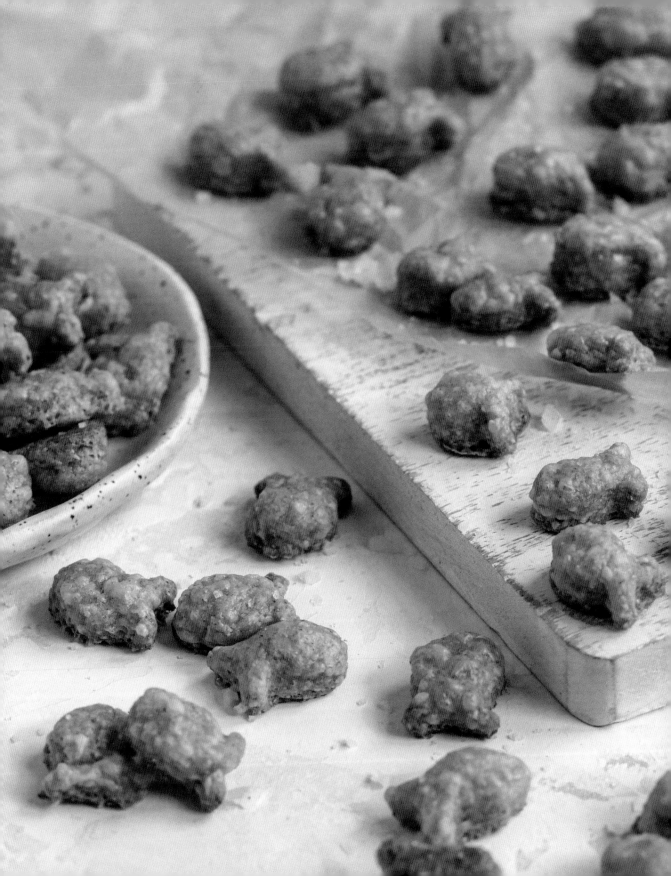

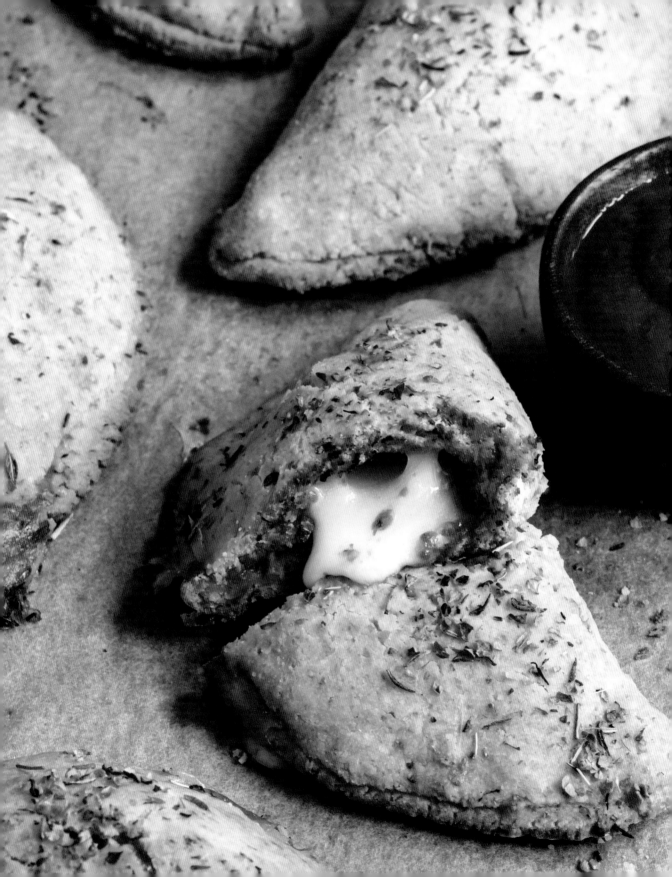

HOMEMADE "HOT POCKETS"

To simplify the prep, I take a little shortcut by using Simple Mills Almond Flour Pizza Dough Mix. Feel free to customize the filling in these with veggies, olives, and cooked meats. Any way you like it!

Makes 8 pockets
Prep Time: 20 minutes
Cook Time: 18 minutes
Total Time: 38 minutes

One 9.8-ounce box Simple Mills Almond Flour Pizza Dough Mix

⅓ cup filtered water

2 tablespoons apple cider vinegar

2 tablespoons extra virgin olive oil

½ cup thick pizza sauce

1 cup shredded mozzarella cheese

¼ cup grated parmesan cheese

Italian seasoning, for topping

Preheat the oven to 350°F.

Combine the pizza dough mix with the water, vinegar, and oil, and mix until a dough has formed, using your hands to squeeze and press the dough together. Let the dough rest for 5 to 10 minutes.

Take roughly ¼ cup of dough in your hands and roll it to form a ball. If the dough seems dry and cracks, sprinkle it with water and squeeze it again to combine. Begin to flatten the dough in your hands. Then place the dough on a parchment-lined baking sheet and continue to flatten it using your fingertips until you have formed an oval roughly 4½ to 5 inches long and about ⅛ inch thick.

Dab 1 tablespoon of pizza sauce in the middle of the flattened dough. Top the sauce with some mozzarella and a sprinkle of Parmesan. Fold one side of the dough over and press and seal the edges with your fingertips. Don't worry if the dough cracks a little on top—just pinch it together or lay a small piece of additional flattened dough over the crack to cover it up.

Repeat with the remaining ingredients to make a total of 8 pockets. Sprinkle the Italian seasoning on top and bake the pockets until they're golden brown, about 18 minutes. Let them cool slightly and serve.

REAL FOOD FRUIT LEATHER

This is a true fruit snack, unlike most that you'll find in stores, which contain hardly any real fruit. Those store-bought fruit snacks are typically full of corn syrup, dyes, and other nasties. And that's why I make these instead. They taste so much better than the packaged variety too—fresh and delicious.

Makes 8 to 10 servings
Prep Time: 10 minutes
Cook Time: 3 hours to 3 hours 30 minutes
Total Time: 3 hours 10 minutes to 3 hours 40 minutes

4 cups fruit of choice
2 tablespoons raw honey
2 teaspoons fresh lemon juice
1 teaspoon vanilla extract

Preheat the oven to 170°F. Line a heavy large baking sheet with parchment paper.

Place all the ingredients in a blender and blend until smooth.

Pour the mixture onto the prepared baking sheet and spread evenly using an offset spatula. You want a thin layer without any holes in it (but don't worry if the parchment wrinkles slightly in a few places).

Place the sheet in the oven and bake the fruit mixture until it is no longer sticky to the touch, about 3 to 3 ½ hours. Let the fruit leather cool completely.

Using scissors, a pizza cutter, or a knife, cut the fruit leather into strips. Roll each strip up in its parchment and tie it with string or seal it with tape. You can store fruit leather in an airtight container for up to 2 weeks.

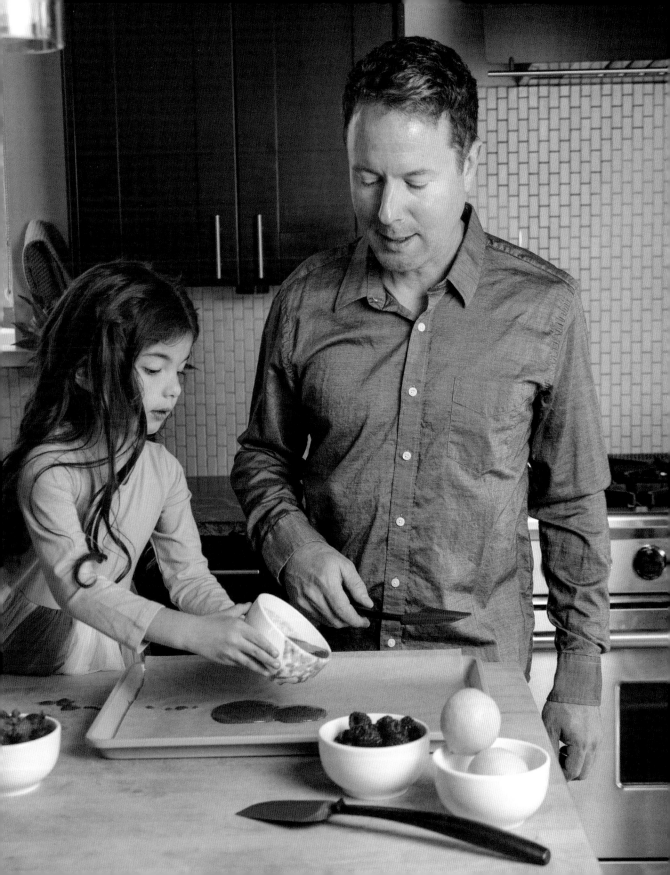

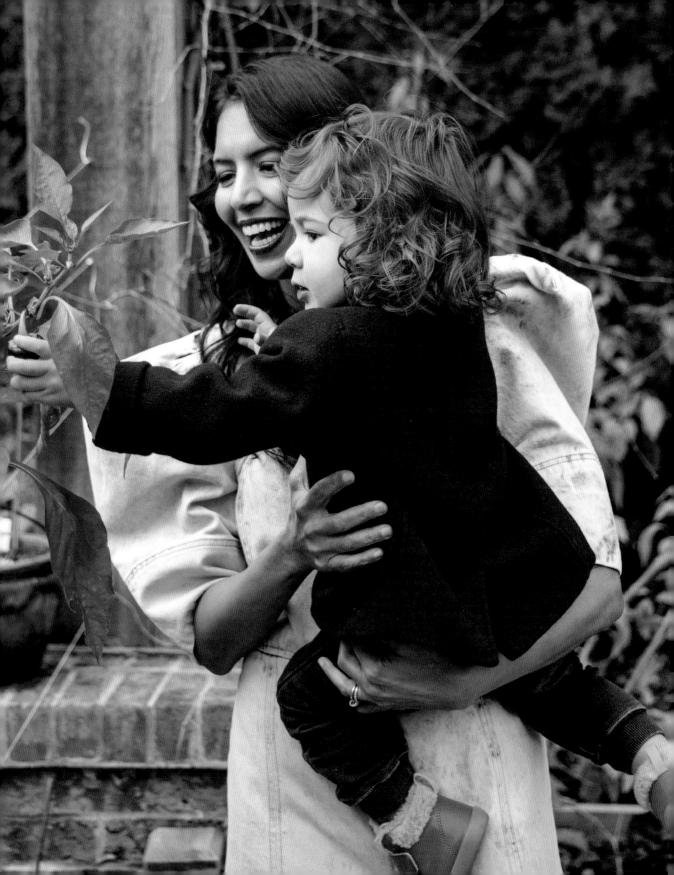

chapter 9

SOUPS AND SALADS

FRESH CHERRY TOMATO & CUCUMBER SALAD

Every time I eat this I feel like a million bucks. It's so refreshing and detoxifying. Next time you need something light to serve with fish or chicken, this salad is the ticket! I love to serve this one with the Meatball Skewers on page 220.

Makes 4 servings
Prep Time: 10 minutes

2 medium cucumbers, diced
1 cup cherry tomatoes, halved
1 shallot, sliced thin
¼ cup chopped fresh parsley
2 tablespoons chopped fresh mint
¼ cup extra virgin olive oil
2 tablespoons lemon juice
2 tablespoon apple cider vinegar
1 teaspoon raw honey
Sea salt and fresh ground black pepper, to taste

Place the cucumbers, tomatoes, shallot, and fresh herbs in a bowl and combine lightly.

In a separate bowl, whisk together the oil, lemon juice, vinegar, and honey. Pour the dressing over the tomato-cucumber mix and toss to combine. Season with salt and pepper and serve.

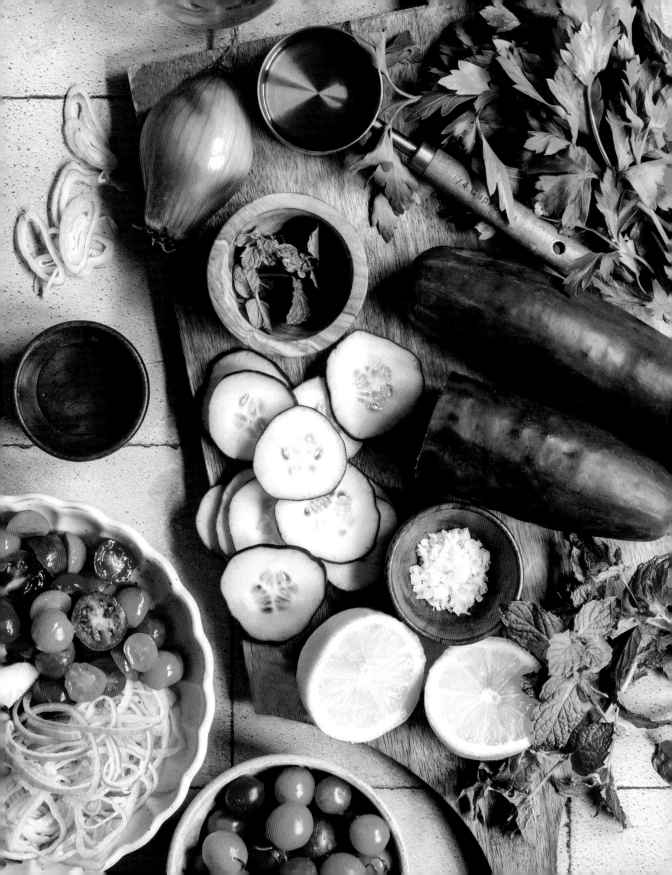

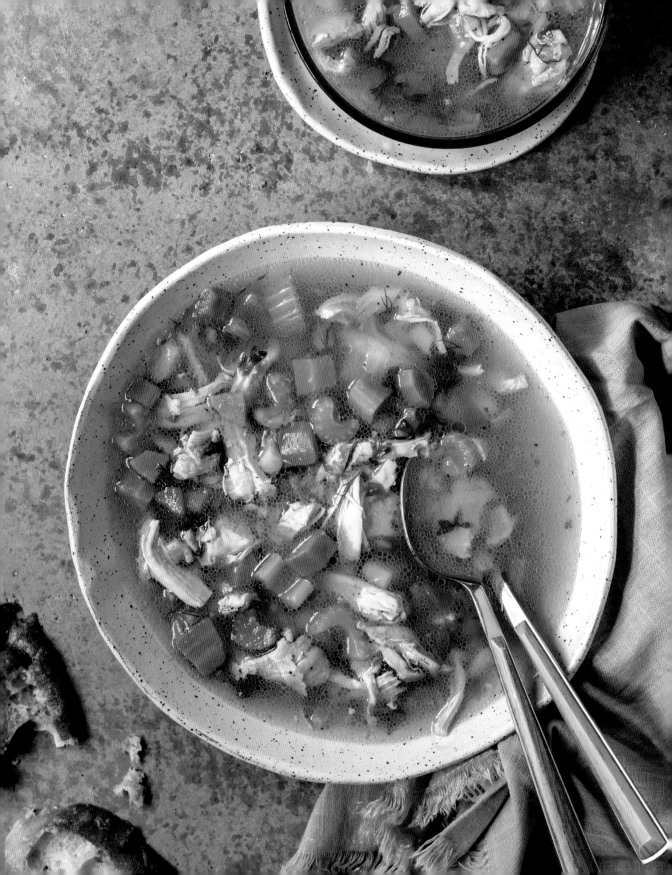

GINGER CHICKEN SOUP

This healing soup is like your favorite warm blanket. It makes for a cozy and comforting meal on a cold day or any time you want the house to feel like home. It's perfect for when anyone in the family is feeling under the weather too—the bone broth, ginger, and vegetables work miracles, I tell ya! If you like a brothy soup, add an additional 2 cups of bone broth. For a heartier meal, serve it with cooked rice or noodles.

Makes 4 servings
Prep Time: 15 minutes
Cook Time: 35 minutes
Total Time: 50 minutes

1 to 2 tablespoons olive oil

1 pound boneless skinless chicken thighs

4 to 5 medium carrots, chopped

2 celery stalks, chopped

1 small yellow onion, diced

1-inch piece fresh ginger root, minced

5 cups low-sodium chicken bone broth

¼ cup chopped fresh parsley

1 tablespoon chopped fresh dill

½ to 1 teaspoon sea salt

½ teaspoon ground black pepper

Heat the oil in a large soup pot over medium-high heat.

Add the chicken thighs and cook them until browned, about 3 minutes per side. Add the carrots, celery, onion, and ginger, and sauté until the vegetables begin to soften, about 5 to 7 minutes.

Add the remaining ingredients and bring to a boil. Reduce the heat to medium-low, cover the pot, and simmer the soup until the chicken is cooked through and the flavors blend, about 20 minutes.

Before serving, break up the chicken.

TOMATO KALE SOUP

I can't even begin to list all the many reasons I love this soup: it's really easy to make, it lasts for a few days, it freezes well, it can feed a crowd, everyone loves it . . . I could go on and on. I take the classic tomato soup up a notch by pureeing in cannellini beans for additional protein and fiber, which also makes it "creamy" without the cream. Serve this with a salad, crunchy crackers, or a slice of toasted sprouted-grain bread.

Makes 4 to 6 servings
Prep Time: 10 minutes
Cook Time: 35 minutes
Total Time: 45 minutes

1 tablespoon olive oil
1 small yellow onion, chopped
4 carrots, peeled and chopped
2 garlic cloves, minced
1 cup filtered water
2 tablespoons chopped fresh basil
1 tablespoon fresh rosemary
1 tablespoon chopped fresh sage
1 bay leaf
1 teaspoon sea salt
½ teaspoon red pepper flakes
¼ teaspoon ground black pepper
24 ounces pureed tomatoes
4 cups vegetable or chicken broth
1 cup cooked cannellini beans
2 cups chopped curly kale

Heat the oil in a large pot over medium heat.

Add the onion and carrots and cook them for 4 to 5 minutes.

Add the garlic and cook the veggies for another 1 to 2 minutes.

Add 1 cup of filtered water along with the remaining ingredients except the kale.

Bring the soup to a boil then reduce to a simmer. Cook it for 25 minutes.

Discard the bay leaf and carefully puree the soup using an immersion or counter blender.

Add the kale to the pureed soup while it's still in the pot and stir it a few times to let the kale wilt. Serve this soup while it's still warm.

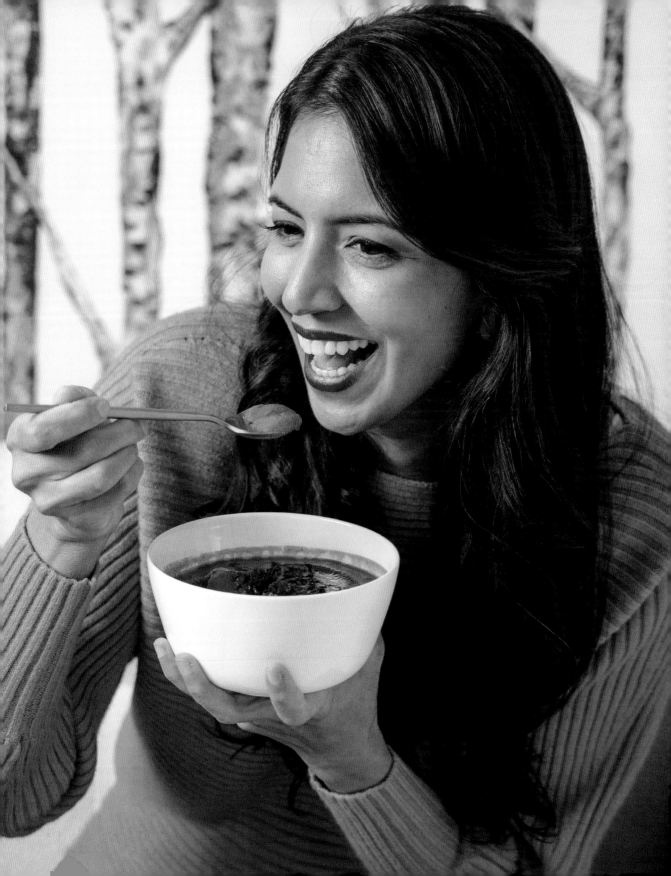

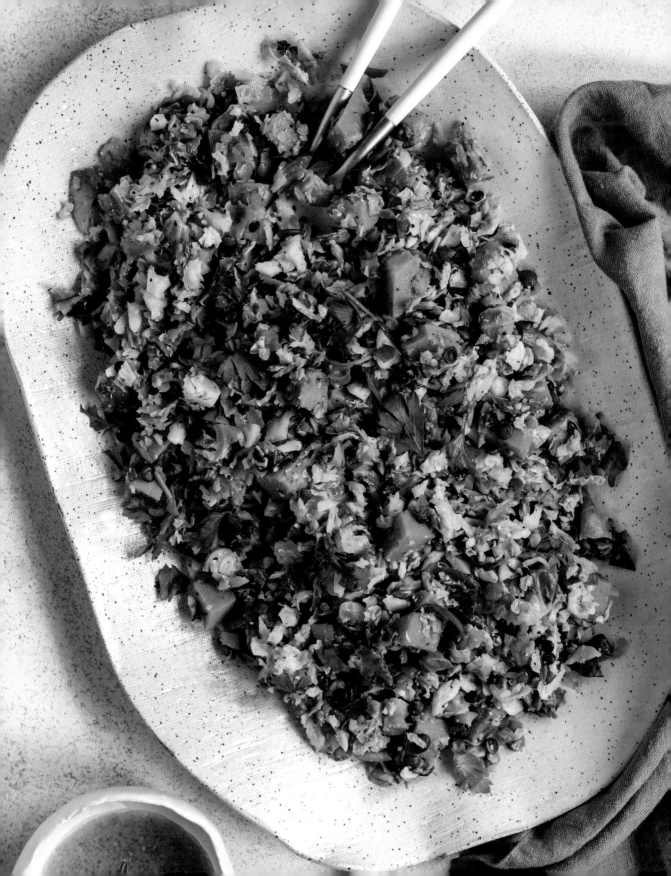

GOOD FORTUNE SALAD

The star ingredient here is one of the most powerful and underappreciated cruciferous vegetables: brussels sprouts. If you've never tried raw brussels sprouts before, you've got to try this salad, because it will make you a lover of them. Remember to shred or cut your brussels sprouts finely for maximum enjoyment. I like to make this salad at the beginning of the year; I named it Good Fortune Salad because lentils are thought to bring good luck in the New Year. May this salad bring you good fortune and health!

Makes 4 servings
Prep Time: 15 minutes
Cook Time: 35 minutes
Total Time: 50 minutes

SALAD

1 butternut squash
1 teaspoon coconut oil
16-ounce bag of brussels sprouts, washed and cleaned
1 cup cooked lentils

DRESSING

1 tablespoon pure maple syrup
1 tablespoon grain mustard
2 tablespoons olive oil
1 tablespoon apple cider vinegar
¼ teaspoon sea salt
Ground black pepper, to taste
½ cup shredded Pecorino Romano cheese (optional)

Preheat the oven to 400°F.

Cut the butternut squash in half and remove the seeds and outer skin. Cut flesh into cubes.

Place the squash cubes on a parchment-lined baking sheet and drizzle with coconut oil. Roast for 30 to 35 minutes or until fork tender.

While the squash is cooking, finely chop the brussels sprouts and make the dressing. To make the dressing, whisk together all the ingredients in a bowl.

To serve, combine the brussels sprouts with the butternut squash and lentils. Top with the dressing and cheese and toss to combine.

STRAWBERRY SPINACH CRUNCH SALAD

This fresh salad is sweet and savory with flavors that POP! It makes an incredible light lunch that's easy to pack for school or work. You can store the dressing and prepped ingredients in your fridge, and then simply assemble it for lunch on busy days. Make sure you keep the dressing on the side until you're ready to eat!

Makes 4 servings
Prep Time: 15 minutes

4 cups mixed greens
3 cups baby spinach
1 cup sliced strawberries
2 avocados, peeled and diced
1 cucumber, thinly sliced
3 radishes, thinly sliced
¼ cup sliced almonds
¼ cup goat feta cheese

Place all of the salad ingredients in a bowl and toss them to combine.

To make the vinaigrette: Whisk together the ingredients. Pour over the salad, toss, and serve.

VINAIGRETTE

½ cup extra virgin olive oil
5 tablespoons apple cider vinegar
1 tablespoon raw honey
2 teaspoons Dijon mustard
1 large shallot, diced
Sea salt and ground black pepper, to taste

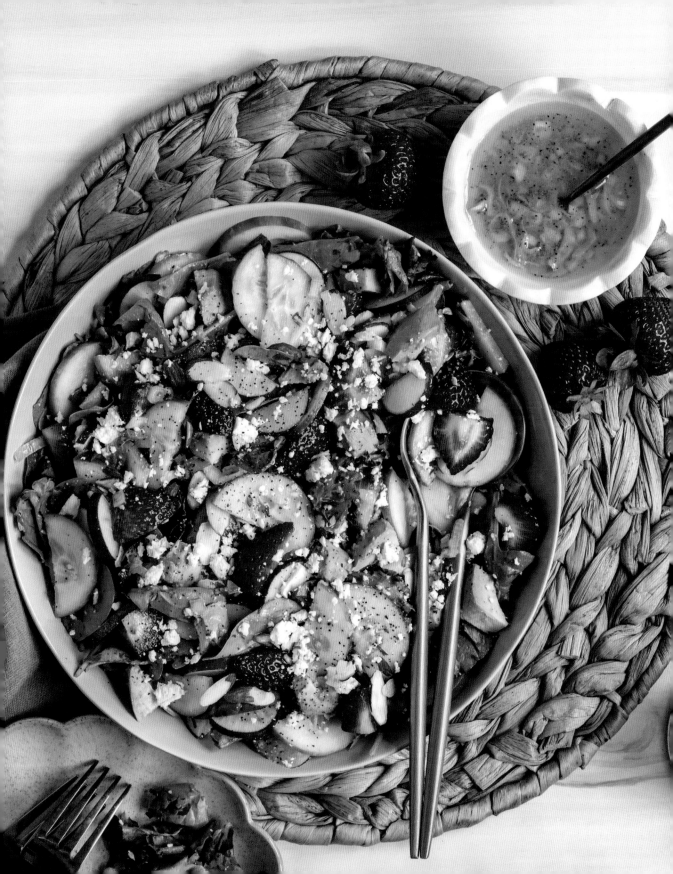

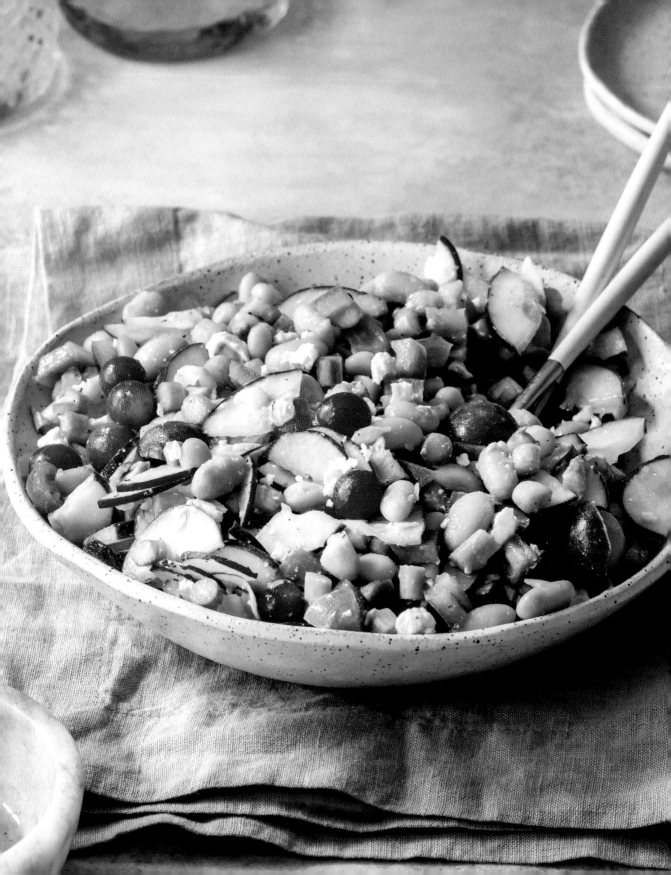

LOADED CANNELLINI BEAN SALAD

This salad is "loaded" with so many tasty vegetables it makes the perfect side dish for just about anything. It's also hearty enough to stand on its own as a light lunch or dinner. I love to make a bowl of this and portion it out into lunch boxes. That way I know my child is getting a hefty variety of veggies along with healthy proteins and fats.

Makes 4 servings
Prep Time: 15 minutes

BEAN SALAD

¼ pound asparagus (6 to 7 stalks), ends trimmed and stems diced
½ cucumber, thinly sliced and halved
1 cup cherry tomatoes, halved
1 green bell pepper, diced
3 radishes, thinly sliced and halved
1 ½ cups cooked cannellini beans
¼ cup crumbled goat feta cheese
¼ cup chopped fresh basil

Place all of the salad ingredients in a bowl and toss to combine.

VINAIGRETTE

¼ cup extra virgin olive oil
2 tablespoons apple cider vinegar
2 tablespoons lemon juice
1 teaspoon Dijon mustard
1 teaspoon pure maple syrup
¼ teaspoon thyme
Sea salt and ground black pepper, to taste

To make the vinaigrette: Whisk together all the ingredients. Pour it over the salad, toss, and serve.

CARROT LENTIL SOUP

My husband and I once ate this soup three nights in a row for dinner. What? Yes, it is THAT good. The sweetness of the carrots—married with the spiciness of the ginger and creaminess of the beans— so freaking yummy. This soup is so supremely satisfying because each serving contains a serving of lentils, which are packed with protein and fiber.

Makes 6 servings
Prep Time: 15 minutes
Cook Time: 38 minutes
Total Time: 53 minutes

1 ½ cups yellow split lentils (alternative: red lentils)

2 teaspoons unrefined virgin coconut oil

1 small yellow onion, diced

6 large carrots, diced

2 garlic cloves, minced

2-inch piece fresh ginger root, minced

1 teaspoon ground cinnamon

alternative: red lentils)

4 cups vegetable or chicken stock

2 tablespoons pure maple syrup

1 bay leaf

1 teaspoon sea salt

¼ teaspoon ground black pepper

2 cups filtered water

Place the lentils in a bowl and cover them with 3 cups of water. Let them soak for at least 8 hours or overnight. Drain the lentils.

Heat the oil in a large pot over medium heat. Add the onion and carrots, and sauté them until the vegetables begin to soften, about 4 to 5 minutes. Add the garlic, ginger, and cinnamon, and sauté the veggies for 2 to 3 minutes more.

Add the soaked, drained lentils, vegetable stock, maple syrup, bay leaf, salt, and pepper to the pot. Mix in 2 cups of filtered water. Bring the soup to a boil, reduce the heat to low, cover the pot, and simmer the soup, stirring it occasionally, until the carrots are very tender and the flavors blend, about 30 minutes.

Remove the bay leaf. Using an immersion or counter blender carefully puree the soup. Ladle it into bowls and serve.

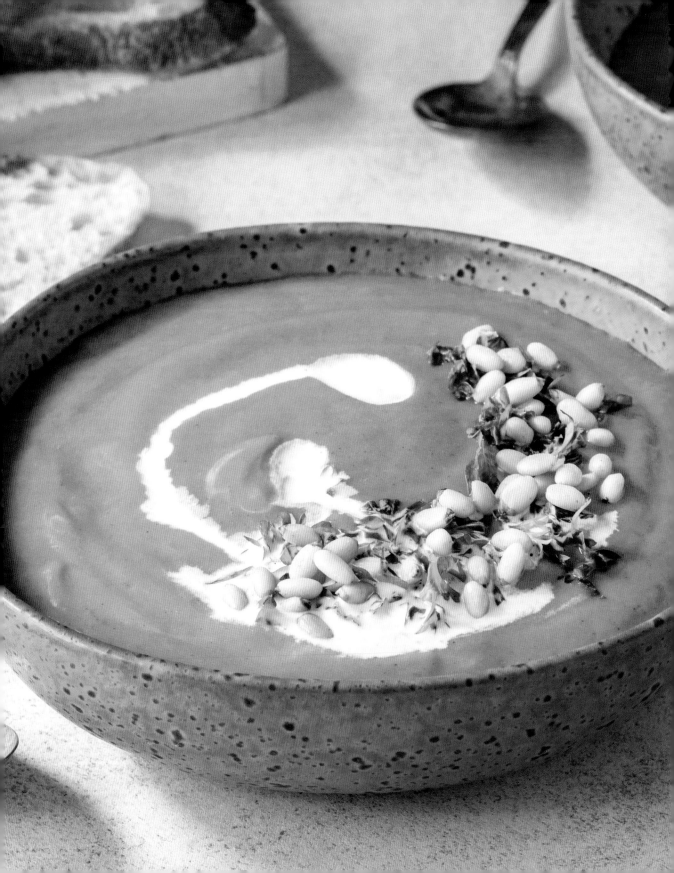

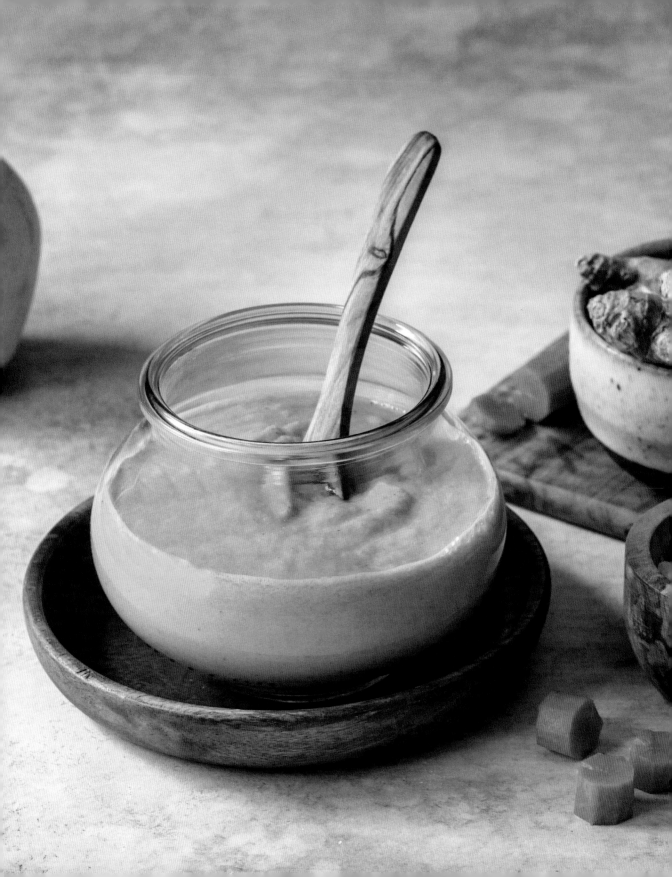

JAPANESE HIBACHI-NIGHT DRESSING

I'll never forget the first time I took my kids to a hibachi restaurant or the amazement on their faces when the chef did the onion "volcano." This salad dressing reminds me of the tangy, miso-based dressing I've had on appetizers at hibachi grills. It's so easy to make: throw everything in a blender and hit go! It's so freaking healthy too without the soybean oil!

Makes 1 ⅔ cup dressing
Prep Time: 10 minutes

1 carrot, trimmed and chopped (about 1 cup)
¼ cup diced white onion
¼ cup chopped fresh ginger root
¼ cup rice wine vinegar
3 tablespoons toasted sesame oil
2 tablespoons white miso paste
2 tablespoons raw honey or coconut sugar
2 tablespoons extra virgin olive oil
½ teaspoon sea salt
¼ teaspoon ground black pepper
¼ cup filtered water

Place all the ingredients in a blender with ¼ cup filtered water. Blend until smooth. Cover and refrigerate the dressing until you are ready to use it. It will keep at least 2 days in the fridge.

ULTIMATE VEGGIE PASTA SALAD

I cringe when I think about the pasta salads I used to buy. You know those pre-made salads from the store with refined-flour pasta and unhealthy soybean oil? Yuck. This homemade pasta salad is a million times better for you. It starts with the best ingredients and packs in the veggies! Serve this when you are cooking out on the grill. Double the recipe to serve at your next get-together with friends and family.

Makes 3 to 4 servings
Prep Time: 10 minutes, plus 20
  to 30 minutes to marinate
Cook Time: 15 minutes
Total Time: 25 minutes

6 ounces lentil pasta
1 small zucchini, sliced thin and halved
½ red bell pepper, diced
1 cup cherry tomatoes, halved
¼ cup diced red onion
3 to 4 radishes, sliced thin
¼ cup chopped parsley

Cook the lentil pasta according to directions on the package.

Once the pasta has cooled and drained, put it in a bowl with the rest of the salad ingredients and mix to combine.

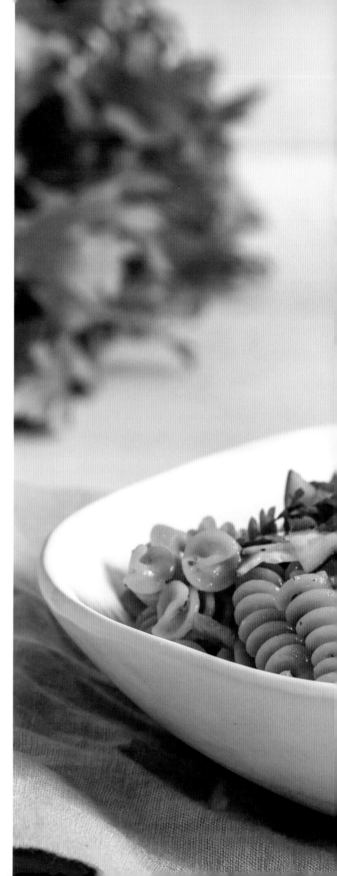

VINAIGRETTE

¼ cup extra virgin olive oil
2 tablespoons apple cider vinegar
1 tablespoon lemon juice
1 garlic clove, minced
1 teaspoon Dijon mustard
1 teaspoon raw honey, more as desired
½ teaspoon oregano
Sea salt and ground black pepper, to taste

To make the vinaigrette, whisk together all the ingredients.

Pour the vinaigrette over the pasta salad and mix well. Let the pasta salad sit for at least 20 to 30 minutes to marinate before serving it.

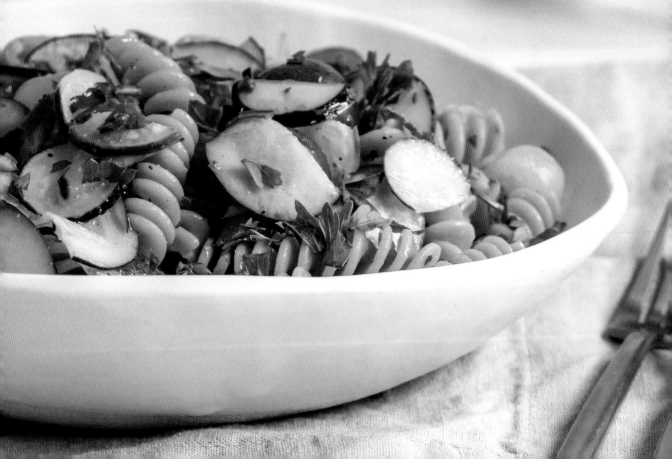

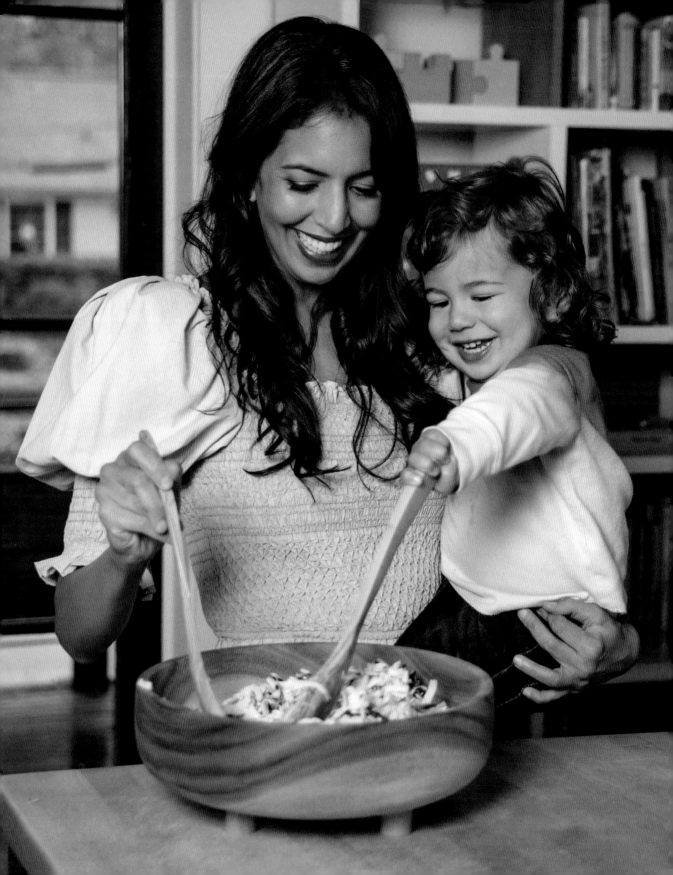

TRI-COLOR COLESLAW

This classic coleslaw is on regular rotation at our house. It packs beautifully in lunch boxes and makes a yummy, crunchy side. I love to serve this coleslaw with simple pulled chicken or the Teriyaki Pork Tenderloin from page 209. Pro Tip: Make sure you check the ingredients on your mayonnaise and try to avoid those made with soybean oil, which is just about every brand out there! The mayo I use is made with avocado oil and organic eggs.

Makes 4 to 6 servings
Prep Time: 15 minutes

2 tablespoons mayo (look for one made with avocado oil)

2 tablespoons apple cider vinegar

2 teaspoons pure maple syrup

½ lemon, juiced

½ teaspoon celery seed

½ small head green cabbage, finely chopped (about 5 cups)

½ small head purple cabbage, finely chopped (about 4 cups)

2 carrots, shredded

Sea salt and freshly ground black pepper, to taste

In a large bowl, whisk together the mayonnaise, vinegar, maple syrup, lemon juice, and celery seed.

Add cabbage and carrots to the dressing and use tongs to toss. Season with salt and pepper to taste.

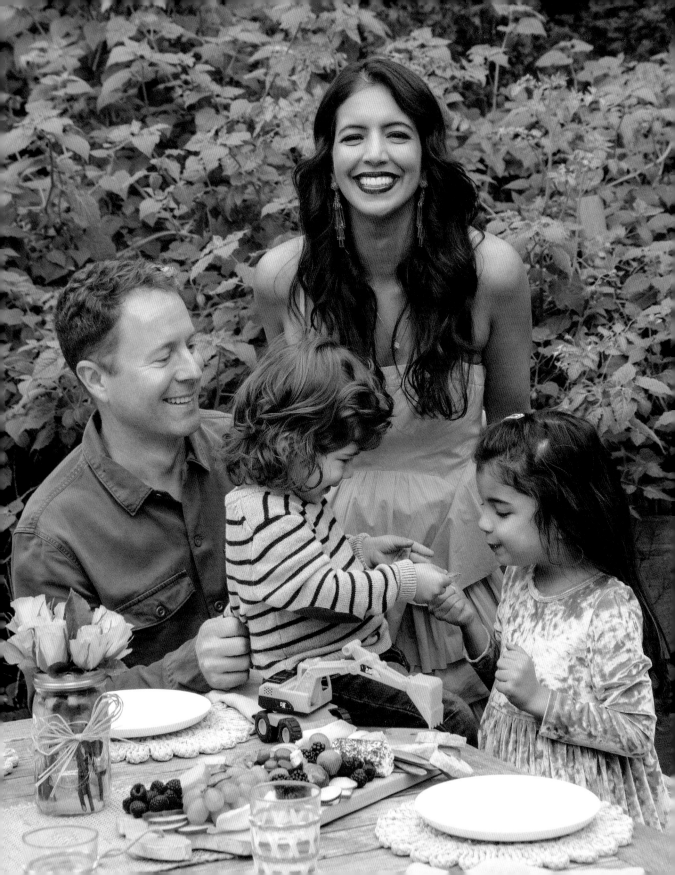

chapter 10

MAINS

TURKEY LETTUCE WRAPS

When I'm craving something fresh and light, these lettuce wraps are one of my go-tos. The crunchy lettuce and jicama paired with saucy Asian turkey is a to-die-for combo! When you want a heartier meal, serve these with the One-Pot Thai-Style Rice on page 251.

Makes 4 servings
Prep Time: 15 minutes
Cook Time: 13 minutes
Total Time: 28 minutes

¼ cup hoisin sauce

2 tablespoons low-sodium tamari

1 tablespoon rice wine vinegar

1 tablespoon chili garlic sauce

2 tablespoons olive oil

2 carrots, shredded

½ small yellow onion, diced

2 garlic cloves, minced

1 tablespoon minced fresh ginger root

1 pound ground turkey

½ small jicama, peeled and diced (1 ½ cups)

16 Bibb, iceberg, or Little Gem lettuce leaves

Optional Toppings

Diced scallions

Chopped cashews

Shredded carrot

In a small bowl, mix together the hoisin, tamari, vinegar, and chili garlic sauce. Set aside.

Heat the oil in a heavy 10-inch skillet over medium heat. Add the carrots and onion, and sauté until softened, about 3 minutes. Add the garlic and ginger, and sauté for an additional minute.

Add the turkey and sauté until it is no longer pink, about 5 minutes.

Add the sauce and jicama. Sauté until the turkey is cooked through, about 4 minutes.

To serve, spoon some of the turkey mixture into each lettuce leaf. Sprinkle with toppings, if desired.

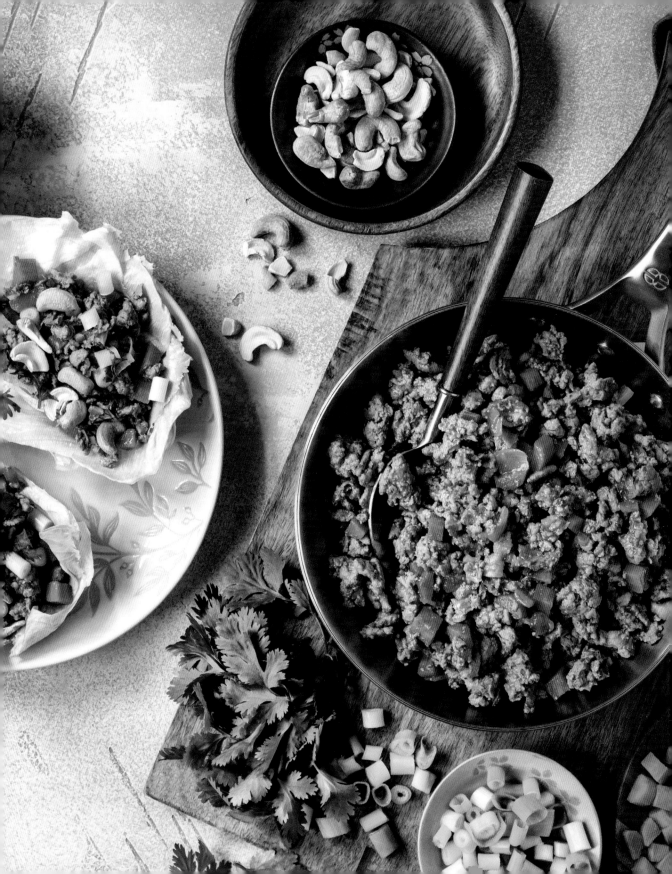

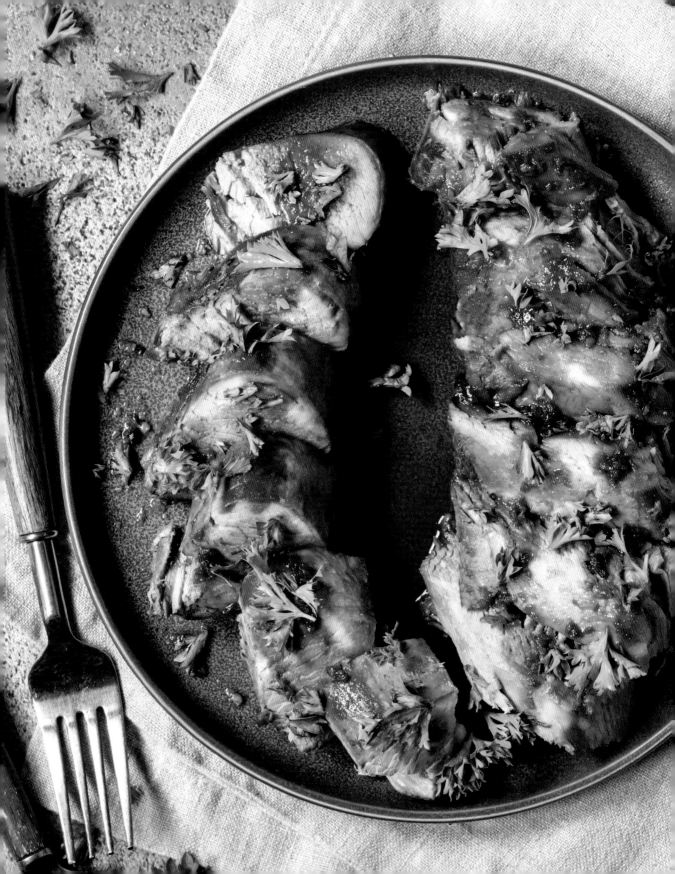

TERIYAKI PORK TENDERLOIN

The 5-minute prep time to make this pork tenderloin is a game-changer on busy days. Pop your tenderloin in the oven with a quick sauce and serve it with a crunchy salad alongside some roasted cauliflower and brown basmati rice. Yum!

Makes 4 servings
Prep Time: 5 minutes
Cook Time: 30 to 35 minutes
Total Time: 35 to 40 minutes

1 ½ pounds pork tenderloin
½ teaspoon paprika
½ teaspoon sea salt
¼ teaspoon ground black pepper
¼ cup raw honey
2 tablespoons low-sodium tamari
2 tablespoons apple cider vinegar
1 tablespoon minced ginger root
2 garlic cloves, minced

Preheat the oven to 350°F.

Place the tenderloin in a baking dish and rub it with paprika, salt, and pepper.

In a small bowl, combine the remaining ingredients. Pour the mixture over the pork.

Bake the tenderloin for 30 to 35 minutes or until the internal temperature reaches 145°F.

Slice the pork in the pan and mix it with the juices before serving.

"CHICK-FIL-A" CHICKEN NUGGETS

Next time you're tempted to hit the drive-thru, I hope you remember you have this recipe for home-made chicken nuggets in your back pocket! These nuggets have that irresistible taste and crispy coating, without the nasty ingredients that fast-food restaurants use. They are also baked, instead of fried, which also makes them a healthier option.

Makes 4 to 6 servings
Prep Time: 10 minutes, plus time to marinate
Cook Time: 15 minutes
Total Time: 25 minutes

2 eggs
¾ cup almond milk
¾ cup pickle juice
3 skinless, boneless chicken breasts, cut into 1-inch pieces
1 ½ cups spelt flour
1 tablespoon powdered sugar
1 teaspoon paprika
½ teaspoon dry mustard
1 teaspoon sea salt
½ teaspoon ground black pepper
2 tablespoons olive oil (in a sprayer)

Preheat the oven to 400°F.

Whisk the eggs, milk, and pickle juice in a bowl. Add the chicken pieces, cover the bowl, and let them marinate in the refrigerator for at least 6 hours (overnight is best).

In a separate bowl, mix together the remaining ingredients except olive oil.

Drain the liquid from the chicken and dredge the pieces in the flour mixture until they are fully coated.

Arrange the chicken pieces on a parchment-lined baking sheet, providing space in between each piece. Spray each piece with olive oil (I like to use a sprayer I fill up myself to avoid chemicals). Bake for 15 to 18 minutes or until they are golden brown and crispy.

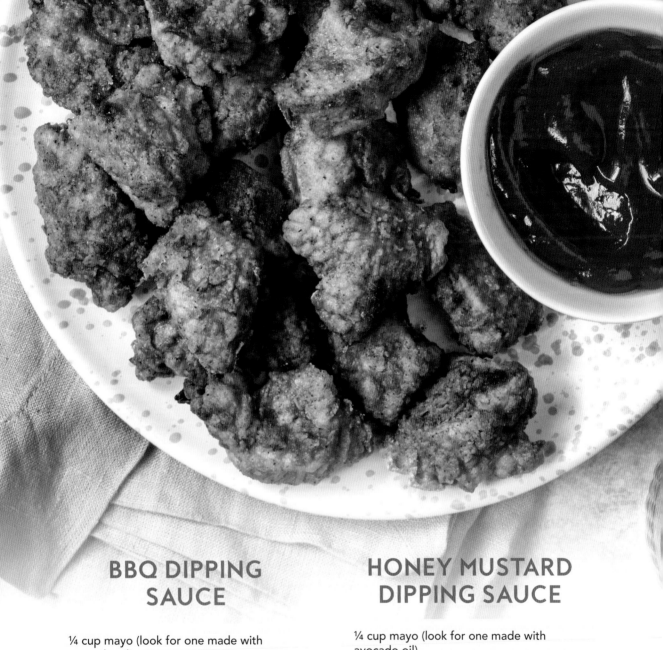

BBQ DIPPING SAUCE

¼ cup mayo (look for one made with avocado oil)

2 tablespoons BBQ Sauce (I like Primal Kitchen Classic BBQ Sauce)

1 tablespoon raw honey

1 tablespoon Dijon mustard

1 tablespoon lemon juice

HONEY MUSTARD DIPPING SAUCE

¼ cup mayo (look for one made with avocado oil)

1 tablespoon Dijon mustard

1 tablespoon raw honey

1 teaspoon apple cider vinegar

Pinch of sea salt

To make each dipping sauce: Combine all the ingredients of your chosen sauce in a bowl and mix them well.

NO NOODLE VEGGIE LASAGNA

The title of this recipe might give you pause, but let me start by saying you will not miss the noodles in this lasagna, I promise! It's gooey, yummy, and so good just like traditional lasagna. Instead of meat, grains, and dairy, though, this lasagna is almost entirely made up of vegetables—a huge win in the nutrition department, if you ask me. This dish also freezes beautifully and is the perfect freezer-to-oven meal when you are short on time.

Makes 6 to 8 servings
Prep Time: 35 minutes
Cook Time: 65 minutes
Total Time: 1 hour 40 minutes

1 tablespoon olive oil
½ yellow onion, diced
2 garlic cloves, minced
24-ounce jar strained tomatoes
1 teaspoon dried basil
½ teaspoon red pepper flakes
½ teaspoon sea salt
15 ounces ricotta cheese
1 egg
1 tablespoon Italian seasoning
1 large zucchini (9 ounces), cut lengthwise into ⅛-inch-thick slices
1 large yellow squash (9 ounces), cut lengthwise into ⅛-inch-thick slices
4 cups lightly packed baby kale or spinach
1 cup shredded goat mozzarella cheese
½ cup shredded raw Parmesan cheese

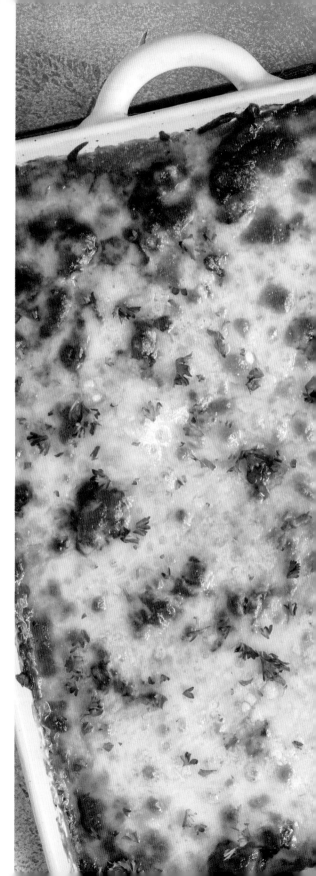

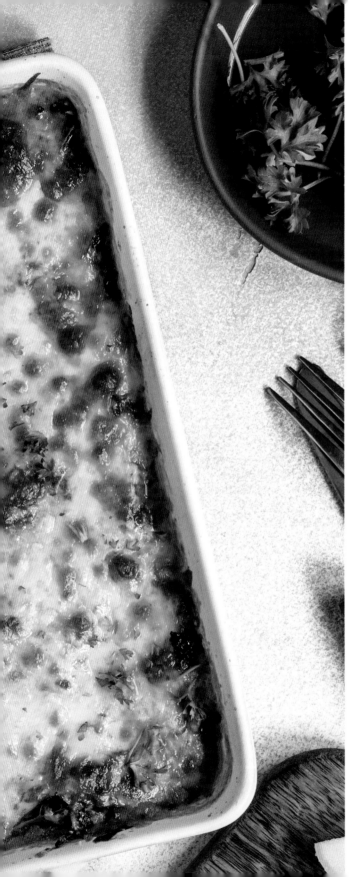

Preheat the oven to 375°F.

Heat the olive oil in a heavy large pot over medium heat. Add the onions and sauté them until they begin to soften, about 4 minutes. Add the garlic and cook for 1 minute.

Add the tomatoes, basil, red pepper flakes, and salt, and bring the mixture to a boil. Reduce the heat to low and simmer the sauce uncovered, stirring it often, until it reduces (3 ¼ cups sauce), about 15 minutes.

In a bowl, mix the ricotta, egg, and Italian seasoning.

Place roughly ⅓ of the cooked tomato sauce (1 cup) on the bottom of a 13 x 9-inch baking dish or pan. Arrange the zucchini in a single layer on top of the tomato sauce. Top with ½ of the ricotta mixture (about 1 cup) in small dollops. Use the back of the spoon to gently and evenly spread the mixture.

Spoon roughly ⅓ more of the tomato sauce (1 cup) over the ricotta; spread it evenly using the back of a spoon. Arrange the yellow squash in a single layer on top of the sauce.

Add the remaining ricotta mixture (about 1 cup) in small dollops and spread it gently and evenly with the back of a spoon.

Arrange the greens on top of the ricotta.

Spoon the remaining tomato sauce (about 1 cup) in dollops over the greens. Sprinkle the mozzarella and Parmesan on top. Cover and bake until bubbly, about 40 minutes. Uncover and bake until the cheese is slightly browned, about 5 minutes. Allow the lasagna to rest for 15 minutes before serving.

If you are reheating this from freezing, preheat the oven to 350 degrees. Bake covered for 30 to 35 minutes or until warmed through.

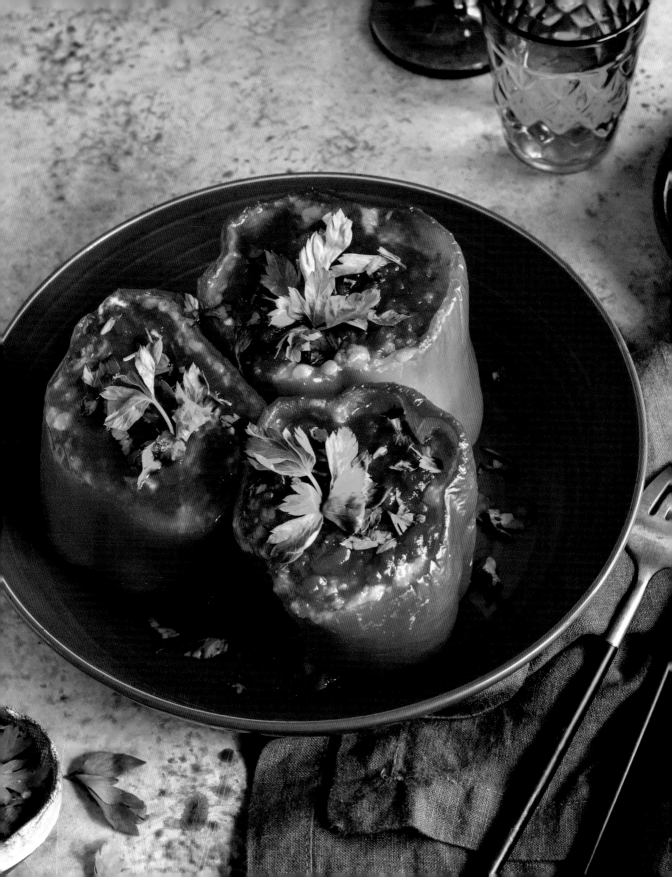

LENTIL STUFFED PEPPERS

I'm always looking for ways to use sprouted lentils in my cooking. They are friendly on your tummy and packed with protein, making them a perfect meatless option to stuff in some gorgeous red peppers. These peppers are delicious, warm, and comforting—and really easy to make after a long day. You could even assemble these ahead of time or make extras so you have leftovers to munch on for a few days.

Makes 4 servings
Prep Time: 20 minutes
Cook Time: 35 minutes
Total Time: 55 minutes

4 large red bell peppers

2 cups lightly packed baby arugula

1 cup sprouted lentils, cooked according to package instructions (about 2 ¼ cups cooked)

1 cup tomato sauce, plus more for topping

½ cup diced yellow onion

3 garlic cloves, minced

2 ounces raw goat cheese, crumbled

½ teaspoon sea salt

¼ teaspoon red pepper flakes

Preheat the oven to 350°F.

Cut off the stem and top of each red pepper. Discard the seeds inside.

Place all remaining ingredients in a bowl and mix to combine.

Fill each red pepper with the lentil mix. Top them off with extra tomato sauce, if desired.

Bake the peppers until they soften slightly and the stuffing is heated through, about 35 minutes. Serve immediately.

MEXICAN CASSEROLE

Whenever my mouth is watering for Mexican food, this healthy dish comes to the rescue! It will satisfy any south-of-the-border craving, without the processed oil and GMO corn found in most restaurant offerings. Make sure to choose organic tortillas to avoid GMO ingredients. My favorite brand, Ezekiel, is found in the freezer section and thaws in just a few minutes on the counter.

Makes 6 to 8 servings
Prep Time: 20 minutes
Cook Time: 45 to 50 minutes
Total Time: 1 hour 10 minutes

1 tablespoon olive oil
1 yellow onion, diced
2 zucchini, diced
1 green bell pepper, diced
1 tomato, diced
1 jalapeño pepper, seeded and minced
2 garlic cloves, minced
1 tablespoon chili powder
1 teaspoon ground cumin
½ sea salt
¼ teaspoon ground black pepper
1 ½ cups cooked black beans
1 ½ cups cooked kidney beans
15 ounces enchilada sauce of choice
12 sprouted corn tortillas
6 ounces goat cheddar cheese, shredded

Optional Toppings

Romaine lettuce
1 lime, sliced
½ cup sour cream or plain yogurt

Preheat the oven to 350°F.

Heat the olive oil in a heavy large skillet over medium-high heat. Add the onion and sauté until it begins to soften, about 3 minutes.

Add the zucchini, green bell pepper, tomato, jalapeño, garlic, spices, salt, and ground pepper; sauté until the vegetables soften, about 7 minutes. Mix in the beans and stir to heat them through.

Pour half the enchilada sauce on the bottom of a 13 x 9-inch baking pan.

Place half of the corn tortillas on top of the sauce, letting them overlap slightly and cutting or tearing them if needed to fit the corners. Spoon half the bean mixture on top.

Repeat, adding another layer of tortillas and then the rest of the bean mixture, ending with the remaining enchilada sauce on top.

Sprinkle with shredded cheese and bake the casserole covered for 30 to 35 minutes. Uncover and bake until it's bubbling, about 5 minutes more.

Let the casserole stand until it's firm enough to cut, about 10 minutes.

Serve with a salad of romaine lettuce, a slice of lime, and a dollop of sour cream or plain yogurt, if desired.

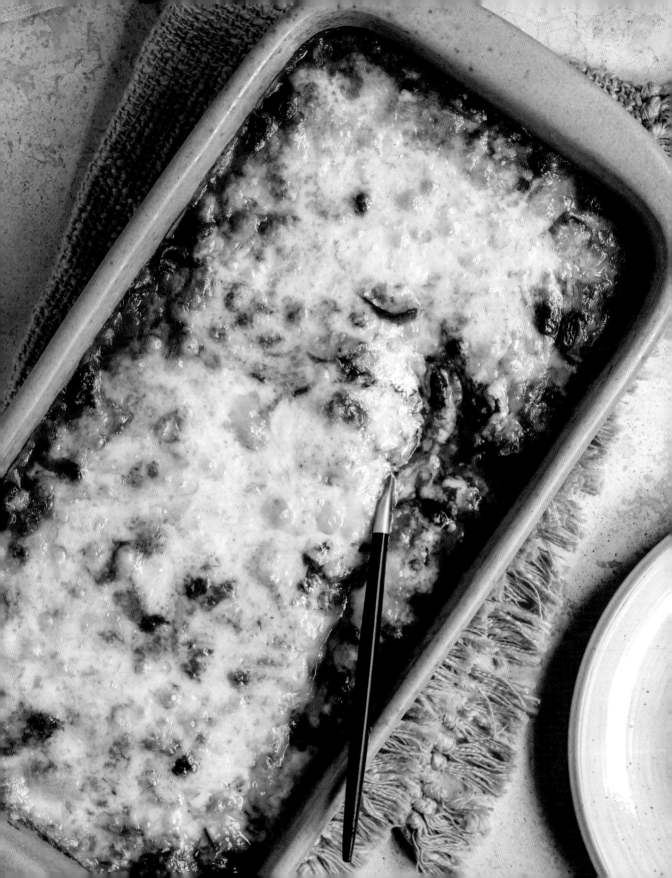

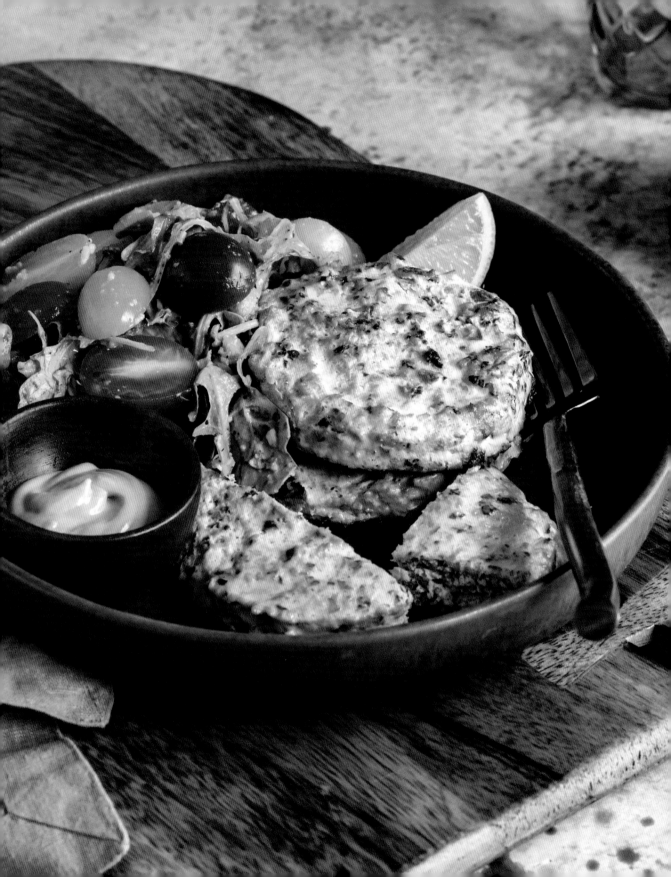

WILD SALMON CAKES
with Arugula Salad

Salmon cakes are really easy to make, and are great for either lunch or dinner. However, I decided to leave out the "cake" part (i.e., the flour). I just don't think using flour is necessary for these bad boys to taste good. And they're . . . phenomenal. Beware that these might become a major hit at your house.

Makes 4 servings
Prep Time: 10 minutes
Cook Time: 15 minutes
Total Time: 25 minutes

1 pound wild salmon, skin removed and diced
¼ cup chopped cilantro
¼ cup chopped parsley
1 egg
1 tablespoon Dijon mustard
¼ teaspoon garlic powder
¼ teaspoon paprika
½ teaspoon sea salt
2 tablespoons chopped red onion
½ lime, juiced
1 to 2 tablespoons olive oil

Preheat the oven to 400°F.

Place all the ingredients for the salmon cakes except the oil in a food processor and pulse until roughly combined. You still want texture, with small to medium-size pieces.

Form the mixture into 4 patties and place them in the refrigerator while you make the salad.

ARUGULA SALAD

1 avocado, peeled and pitted
½ lime, juiced
Sea salt and ground black pepper, to taste
6 cups arugula
1 cup cherry tomatoes, halved

In a large bowl, mash the avocado and lime juice until well combined, and season with salt and pepper.

Add the arugula and mix it in well, making sure all leaves are covered. Add the cherry tomatoes and toss to combine. Set aside.

Place the salmon cakes on a parchment-lined baking sheet. Rub them with oil and place the sheet in the oven. Cook for 12 to 15 minutes or until they are cooked through and flake easily with a fork.

To serve, place some of the arugula salad on a plate and top it with 1 to 2 salmon cakes.

MEATBALL SKEWERS

These skewers are fun for little hands to hold and dip into the hummus. (You can break off the pointy end of the skewer if you are worried someone is going to stab themself.) You can also serve these meatballs in a sandwich; try tucking them inside pita bread with a little hummus. Pair this dish with the Fresh Cherry Tomato & Cucumber Salad on page 184.

Makes 4 servings
Prep Time: 15 minutes
Cook Time: 15 minutes
Total Time: 30 minutes

1 pound ground turkey

¼ cup chopped yellow onion

2 garlic cloves, minced

¾ teaspoon sea salt

½ teaspoon ground black pepper

½ teaspoon red pepper flakes

Bamboo skewers (soaked at least 30 minutes) or stainless steel skewers

2 yellow onions, cut into 2-inch wedges

Olive oil (for brushing)

1 cup hummus of choice

Preheat a grill to 400°F.

Place the turkey, chopped onion, garlic, salt, pepper, and red pepper flakes in a bowl and mix them well. Use 1 tablespoon of mixture to make each mini meatball.

Slide 1 meatball on a skewer and then thread 2 onion pieces. Repeat 2 more times. Continue with the remaining skewers until you have used up all the meatballs.

Brush the skewers with olive oil and grill them for 6 to 7 minutes. Flip them and grill for an additional 7 minutes or until the meatballs are cooked through.

To serve, spread ¼ cup hummus on the center of each plate. Top with meatball skewers. Enjoy!

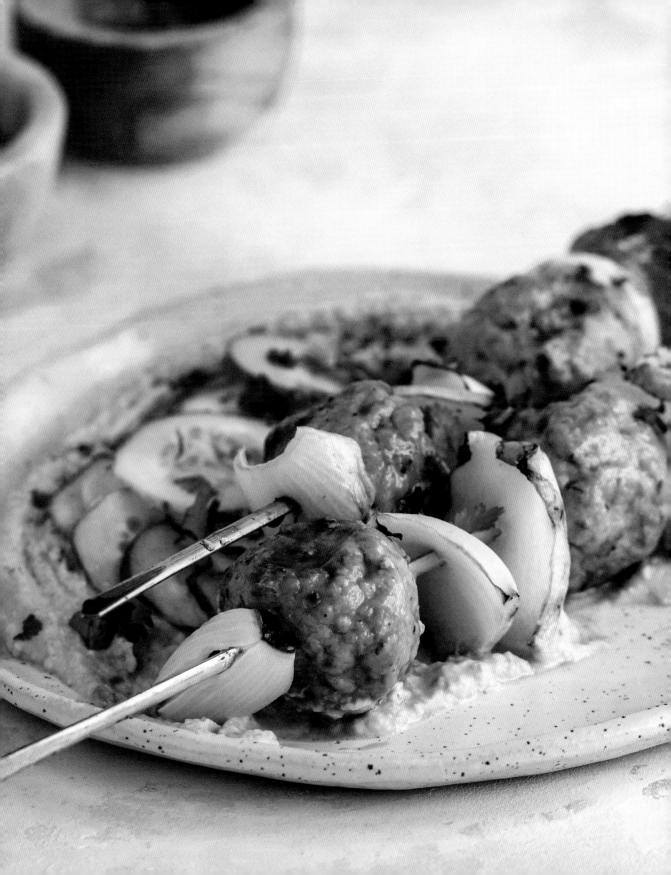

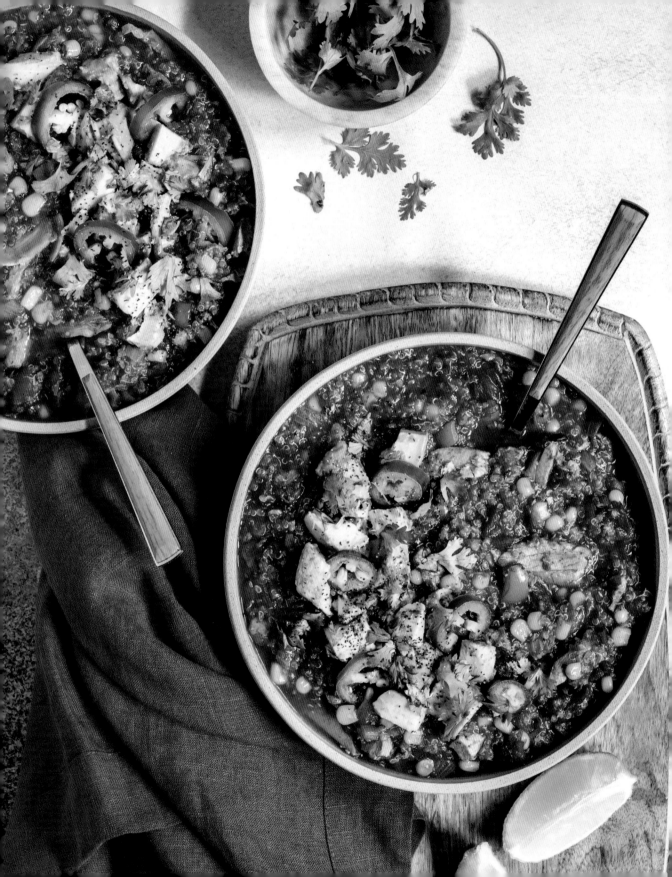

EASY CHICKEN QUINOA CHILI

My secret ingredient in this hearty chili is quinoa. This is a gluten-free seed that contains about 8 grams of protein and 5 grams of fiber per cup. It's also a good source of manganese and magnesium, which is why I love adding quinoa to my meals to bump up the nutritional content. Quinoa has a texture similar to rice and adds a special touch to this chili!

Makes 4 servings
Prep Time: 15 minutes
Cook Time: 35 minutes
Total Time: 50 minutes

2 tablespoons olive oil

5 boneless, skinless chicken thighs

1 medium yellow onion, diced

1 green bell pepper, diced

2 cloves garlic, minced

½ jalapeño, seeded and minced

1 cup quinoa, rinsed

2 cups chicken stock

1 cup cooked black beans

1 cup sweet corn

28-ounce jar diced roasted tomatoes

1 tablespoon chili powder

1 ½ teaspoons ground cumin

1 teaspoon sea salt

¼ teaspoon ground black pepper

Optional Toppings

Lime wedges

Organic cheddar cheese

Sprouted-grain corn chips

Heat the oil in a large pot over medium-high heat. Add the chicken thighs and cook for 3 to 4 minutes per side or until browned. Take them out of the pot and set them aside.

Add the onion, bell pepper, garlic, and jalapeño to the pot and cook for 3 to 4 minutes to soften the vegetables.

Add the quinoa and cook it for 1 minute. Add the chicken stock to deglaze the pan, stirring to release any browned bits from the bottom of the pot.

Add the remaining ingredients and the chicken and bring to a boil. Turn the heat down to a simmer, cover, and cook for 30 to 35 minutes.

Remove the chicken from the pot and shred. Place the chicken back in the pot and mix to combine. Serve with desired toppings.

LEMON ROSEMARY CHICKEN
with Root Vegetables

Everyone who has tried this chicken dish loves it and finds it extremely satisfying. I love making it too, because it comes together in one pan, so I don't have to worry about multitasking. This is one of those meals you can throw together while chatting with your family without missing a beat!

Makes 4 servings
Prep Time: 15 minutes
Cook Time: 40 minutes
Total Time: 55 minutes

2 tablespoons olive oil, divided
1 teaspoon fresh rosemary leaves
1 teaspoon fresh oregano
¼ teaspoon red pepper flakes
2 garlic cloves, minced
1 lemon, juiced
6 boneless, skinless chicken thighs
Sea salt and ground black pepper
½ yellow onion, diced
3 cups diced root vegetables, such as turnips, sweet potatoes, or parsnips
½ cup chicken stock
2 lemons, cut in half
2 sprigs fresh rosemary

Preheat the oven to 400°F.

Place 1 tablespoon olive oil in a bowl with the rosemary leaves, oregano, red pepper flakes, garlic, and lemon juice. Mix to combine.

Sprinkle the chicken with salt and pepper. Add the chicken to the bowl with the spice mix and rub to coat evenly. Set aside.

Heat the remaining 1 tablespoon of oil in a 12-inch cast-iron skillet over medium-high heat. Add the onion and root vegetables and sauté until the vegetables begin to brown, about 7 minutes. Transfer the vegetables to a bowl.

Place the chicken thighs in the pan and cook them over high heat until brown, about 4 minutes per side. Spoon the root vegetables into the skillet around the chicken. Add the chicken stock, lemon wedges, and rosemary sprigs. Place the skillet in the oven and roast everything until the chicken is cooked through and the vegetables are tender, about 25 minutes.

To serve, squeeze some of the lemon wedges over the chicken and vegetables.

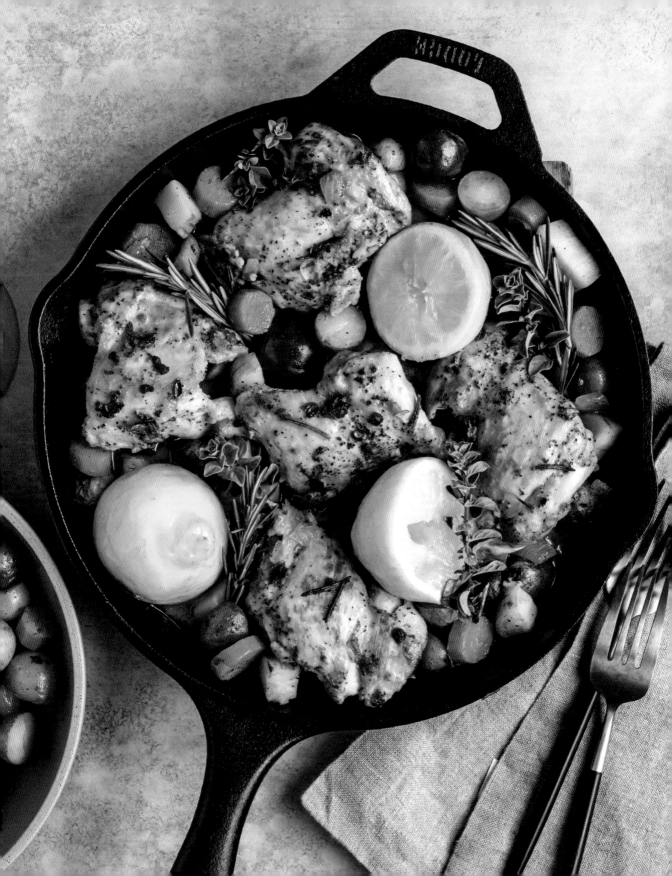

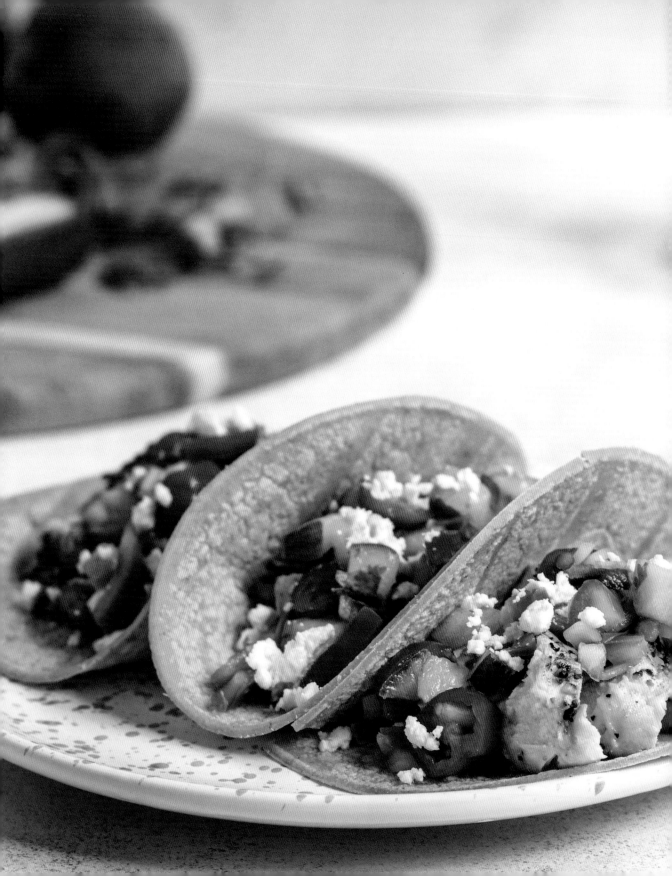

GRILLED CHICKEN TACOS
with Peach Salsa

It's no secret that I love Mexican food. I'm always looking for ways to make it healthier at home because at most restaurants it's made with refined oils, GMO corn, and factory-farmed conventional meats. These homemade chicken tacos cook up quick, and kids love them. Simply grill some pastured chicken and top it with fresh peach salsa and feta, and wrap it up in sprouted corn tortillas. Delish!

Makes 4 servings
Prep Time: 15 minutes
Total Time: 15 minutes

2 large chicken breasts, grilled and sliced
8 to 12 sprouted corn tortillas, warmed
½ cup goat feta cheese

To assemble, take a tortilla and lay 2 to 3 pieces of chicken down the center. Top with the peach salsa and feta cheese.

PEACH SALSA

2 peaches, pitted and diced
½ cup diced red onion
1 cup halved cherry tomatoes
1 green bell pepper, diced
1 jalapeño, seeded and diced
½ cup chopped cilantro
1 to 2 limes, juiced
Sea salt and ground black pepper, to taste

To make the salsa, place all the ingredients in a bowl and mix well.

QUICK AND EASY HOME-BAKED PIZZA

I have a feeling this pizza will become a staple in your household, like it has in mine. The freshness of the ingredients makes it way more satisfying than any frozen pizza. When I suggest making pizza for dinner, I usually hear a big "OH YEAH!" from my husband. When I make these personal pizzas for other family members or friends, they immediately request the recipe. To get your children involved, set out the toppings buffet style and let everyone create their own pizzas before popping them in the oven.

Makes 1 personal-size pizza
Prep Time: 5 minutes
Cook Time: 10 minutes
Total Time: 15 minutes

1 large Ezekiel Sprouted Wheat Tortilla, thawed

4 tablespoons tomato sauce

1 garlic clove, minced

¼ cup chopped yellow onion

¼ cup chopped green bell pepper

¼ cup chopped broccoli florets

5 black olives, sliced

1 ounce goat mozzarella cheese (optional)

½ ounce raw Parmesan cheese (optional)

Crushed red pepper flakes, for sprinkling

Preheat the oven to 450°F.

Place the tortilla on a large parchment-lined baking sheet and put in the oven for 3 to 4 minutes to allow the crust to harden a bit. Once the tortilla has started to slightly crisp along the edges, remove it from the oven.

Place the tomato sauce and garlic on the crust. Top with onion, bell pepper, broccoli, olives, and cheese, being careful not to overload the crust. Return the loaded pizza to the oven and bake for 10 minutes or until the cheese is bubbly.

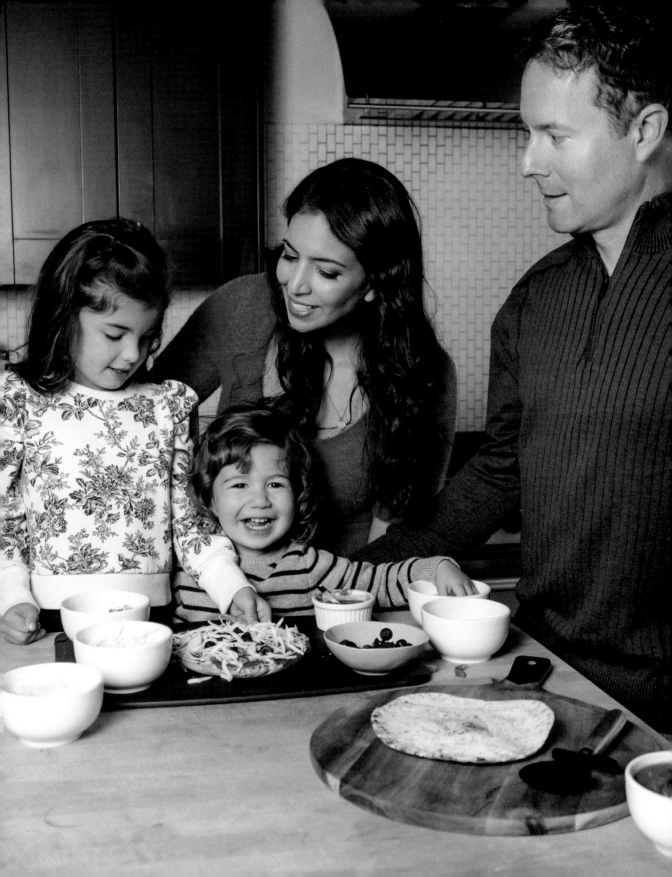

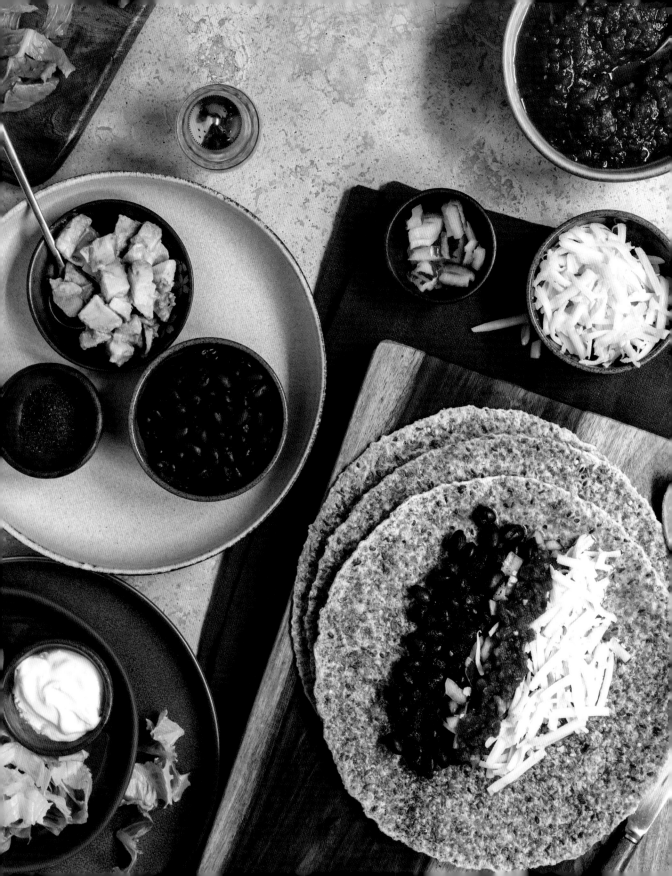

FAST-FOOD BURRITO

These burritos come together FAST with a few amazing store-bought ingredients. That's right: you don't have to make everything from scratch. I can have a fresh burrito ready in a matter of minutes or pull a pre-made one from the freezer (if I am lucky and my husband hasn't eaten the whole stash!). It takes me less than 7 minutes to make 6 of these burritos. Can you beat my time? Ready, set, go!

Makes 6 small burritos
Prep Time: 10 minutes
Cook Time: 10 minutes
Total Time: 20 minutes

6 small Ezekiel Sprouted Grain Tortillas, thawed

One 15-ounce can cooked black beans, drained and rinsed

Chili powder, to taste

½ red onion, sliced thin

2 cups salsa of choice

3 ounces of goat cheddar cheese, shredded

Optional Toppings

Avocado

Romaine lettuce

Sour cream

Lime wedges

Preheat the oven to 375°F.

Place the tortillas on a baking sheet lined with aluminum foil and parchment paper. (This is an important step—you don't want your food to stick to the aluminum foil.)

Spoon ¼ cup of black beans onto each tortilla. Sprinkle chili powder on top of the black beans. Add 1 tablespoon of sliced onion and 1 tablespoon of salsa.

Add ¼ cup cheddar cheese. Roll and wrap each tortilla tightly. Place the sheet in the oven and cook for 10 minutes.

Serve with avocado, romaine, sour cream, lime wedges, and/or more salsa.

MEXICAN-STYLE BAKED ZUCCHINI BOATS

Zucchini is one of my favorite versatile vegetables. You can spiralize it into noodles, make baked goodies, and even make chips out of it! Here's a new twist that maybe you haven't tried before: stuffing zucchini with a tasty taco filling and baking it in the oven. This dish is packed with lots of veggies and so incredibly flavorful. Save this taco seasoning recipe for any time you're making tacos—there's no need to ever buy processed packets again!

Makes 4 servings
Prep Time: 25 minutes
Cook Time 38 minutes
Total Time: 1 hour 3 minutes

ZUCCHINI BOATS

2 very large zucchini
(about 11 ounces each)
1 tablespoon olive oil
1 small yellow squash, diced
½ yellow onion, diced
½ red bell pepper, diced
½ pound ground turkey
2 tablespoons Homemade Taco Seasoning
1 egg, beaten

HOMEMADE TACO SEASONING

1 tablespoon chili powder
1 ½ teaspoons ground cumin
1 teaspoon paprika
1 teaspoon garlic powder
½ teaspoon onion powder
½ teaspoon dried oregano
½ teaspoon sea salt
¼ teaspoon freshly ground black pepper

Preheat the oven to 400°F.

Mix all the taco seasoning ingredients in a bowl and set it aside.

Use a large knife to cut each zucchini lengthwise in half. Using a melon baller or small spoon, carefully scoop out the insides, leaving a ¼- to ⅓-inch-thick shell to make room for the filling.

Heat the oil in a heavy large skillet over medium heat. Add the yellow squash, onion, and bell pepper and sauté until the vegetables begin to soften, about 3 minutes. Add the turkey and 2 tablespoons of taco seasoning and sauté until the turkey is cooked through, about 5 minutes. Remove the skillet from the heat and let the taco filling cool a bit.

When cool, add the beaten egg and mix well. Stuff each zucchini with some of the filling, mounding it slightly and then pressing gently to compact it. Place the boats in a baking pan and bake them uncovered until the zucchini is just tender, about 25 to 30 minutes.

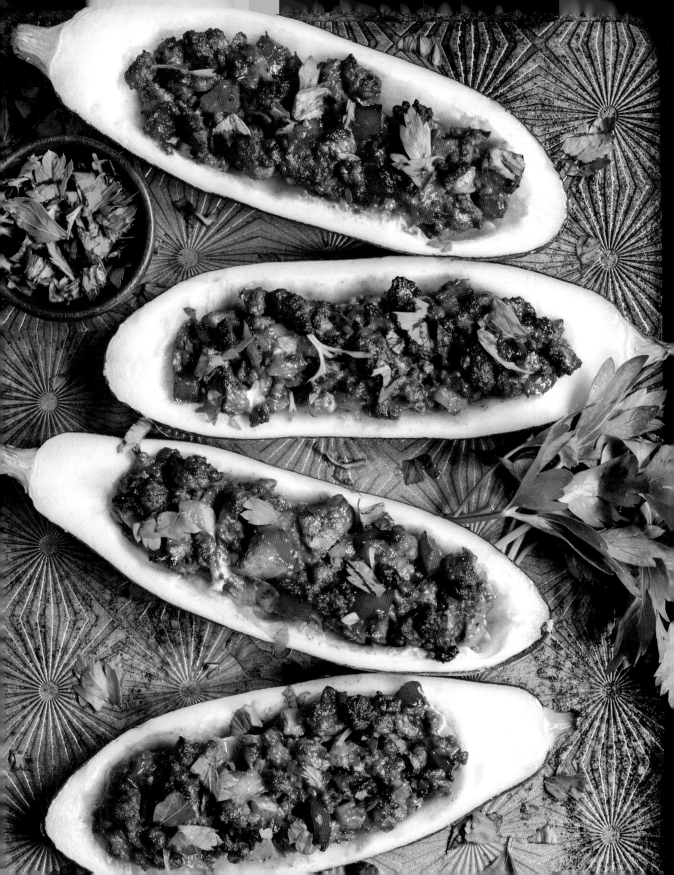

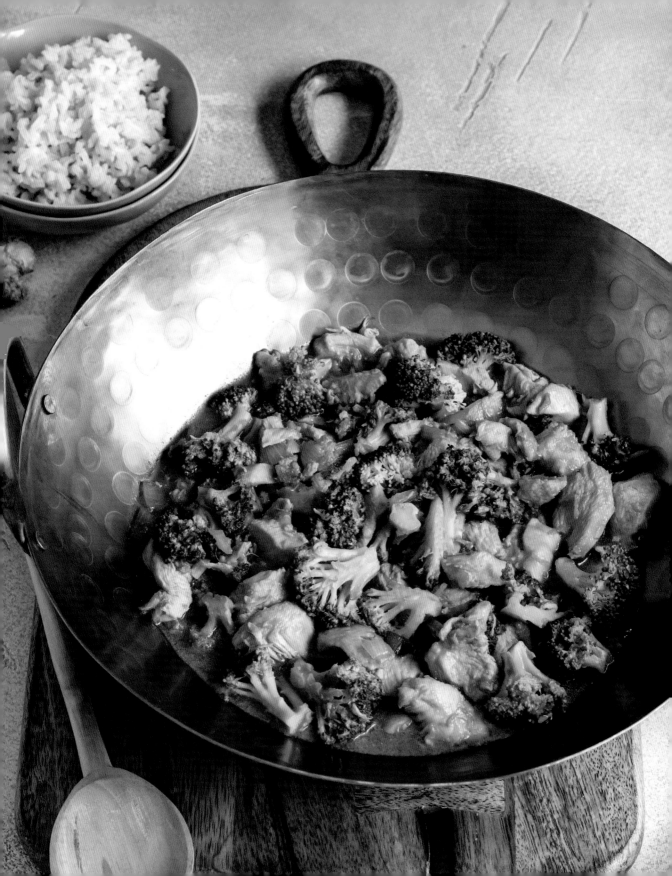

NO FUSS GINGER CHICKEN STIR-FRY

with Broccoli

This stir-fry comes together quickly on busy weeknights. It's savory and so delicious when served over steamed basmati rice or sprouted quinoa. Feel free to switch up the vegetables depending on what you have on hand; but whatever you do, don't skip the ginger! This ingredient is the star in this meal.

Makes 4 servings
Prep Time: 15 minutes
Cook Time 12 minutes
Total Time: 27 minutes

1 pound boneless skinless chicken breasts, cut into 1-inch pieces

2 tablespoons arrowroot powder

¼ cup low-sodium tamari or coconut aminos

2 tablespoons mirin

1 teaspoon toasted sesame oil

1 to 2 tablespoons olive oil

½ yellow onion, diced

2 garlic cloves, minced

1 tablespoon minced fresh ginger root or 1 teaspoon ground ginger

3 cups small broccoli florets, large ones cut in half

¼ teaspoon sea salt, or more to taste

1 cup filtered water

2 cups cooked basmati rice

In a small bowl, coat the chicken cubes in the arrowroot powder. Set aside.

In a separate bowl, mix together the tamari, mirin, and sesame oil. Set aside.

Heat the olive oil in a wok or heavy large skillet over medium-high heat. Add the onion, garlic, and ginger, and sauté until the onion begins to soften, about 3 minutes. Add the chicken and cook it until it is no longer pink, about 5 minutes.

Add the broccoli, tamari sauce, salt, and filtered water. Stir-fry until the chicken is cooked through, the broccoli is crisp-tender, and the sauce begins to thicken, about 4 minutes.

Serve over basmati rice.

CHICKEN AND BLACK BEAN QUESADILLAS

These are so fun to make with older kids. Let them help you shred the cheese and chicken, and then carefully add the fillings to the tortillas. And when they're old enough, they can even get in there and flip! This teaches them so many skills in the kitchen. Cut your quesadillas into triangles with a pizza cutter and dunk them into guac and salsa. The best family dinner night!

Makes 4 servings
Prep Time: 10 minutes
Cook Time: 20 to 29 minutes
Total Time: 35 minutes

3 tablespoons olive oil, divided

1 yellow onion, diced

1 green bell pepper, diced

1 red bell pepper, diced

1 teaspoon chili powder

Sea salt and ground black pepper, to taste

1 cup cooked black beans

1 cup cooked shredded chicken

8 Organic Bread of Heaven flour tortillas or tortillas of choice

2 to 3 cups shredded goat cheddar cheese

Optional Toppings

fresh salsa

guacamole

Heat 2 tablespoons of oil in a sauté pan over medium heat. Add the onion, bell peppers, and chili powder. Cook until tender, about 4 to 5 minutes. Season with salt and pepper.

Take the pan off the heat and add the black beans and cooked chicken. Mix to combine.

In a separate sauté pan, heat the remaining tablespoon of oil over medium-low heat. Add one of the tortillas to the pan and top with ¼ cup shredded cheese. Add ½ cup of the chicken mixture and another ¼ cup of cheese, spreading evenly over the tortilla. Top with another tortilla and let cook until golden brown, about 2 to 3 minutes. Flip the quesadilla and cook for an additional 2 to 3 minutes or until golden brown. Serve with fresh salsa or guacamole.

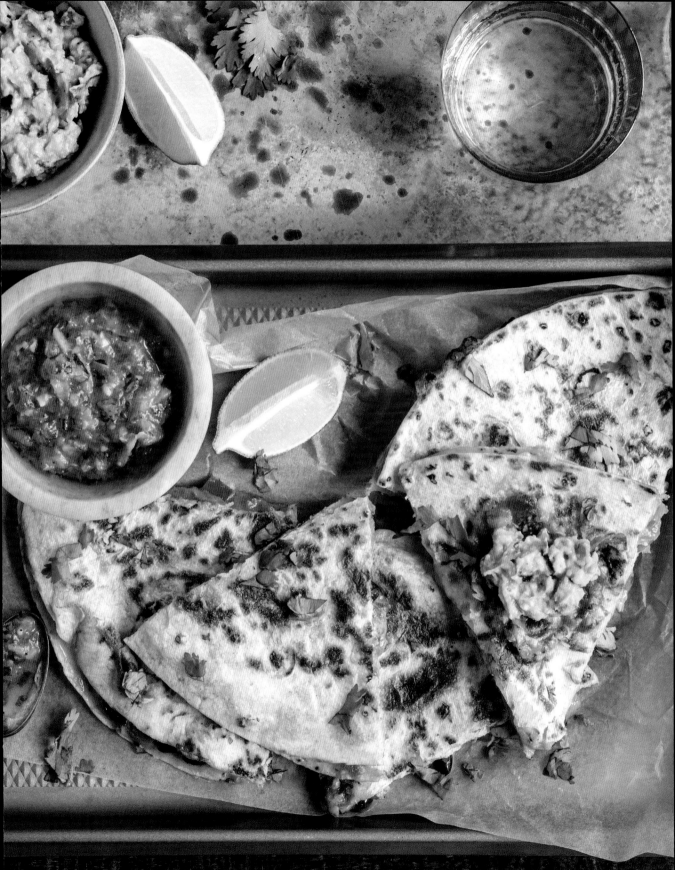

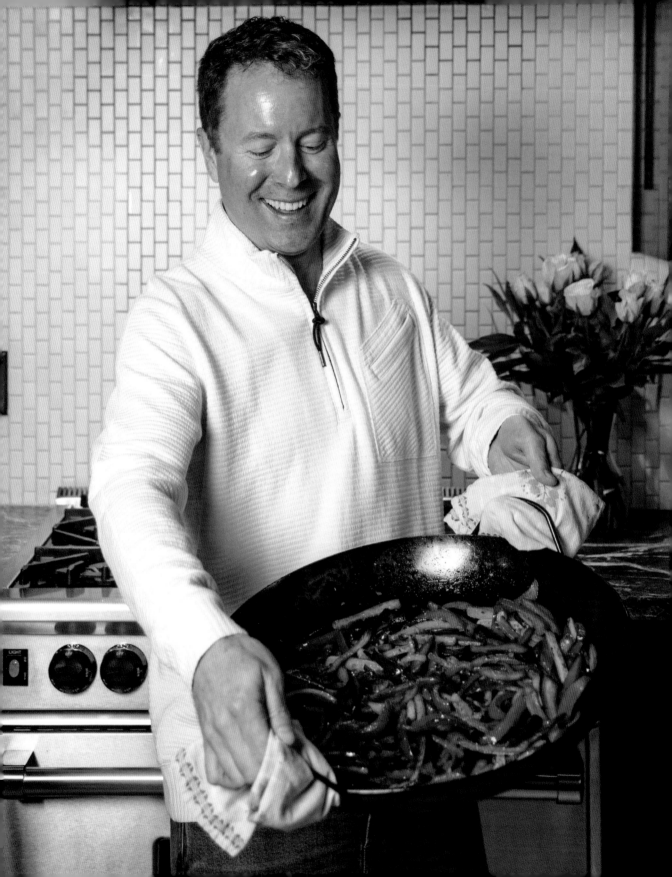

VEGGIE FAJITAS

My mouth is watering just thinking about these. Don't let the simplicity of these fajitas fool you. They're extremely versatile and a great way to get anyone in your house to eat more veggies. I sometimes like to add in shredded chicken, beans, avocado slices, goat-milk cheddar cheese, or olives. Tuck everything inside sprouted corn tortillas or, my current favorite, delicious tortillas made by Organic Bread of Heaven. Dreamy!

Makes 4 servings
Prep Time: 15 minutes
Cook Time: 12 to 15 minutes
Total Time: 30 minutes

2 to 3 tablespoons olive oil
2 red bell peppers, sliced
2 green bell peppers, sliced
1 red onion, sliced thin
1 zucchini, julienned
1 yellow squash, julienned
1 teaspoon sea salt
1 to 2 teaspoons chili powder

Optional Toppings and Accompaniments

Tortillas

Guacamole

Sour cream

Lime wedges

Shredded cheese

Cooked beans

Shredded chicken

Heat the oil on a large fajita pan or skillet over medium heat. Add the veggies and spices and cook until tender.

Serve with the accompaniments as desired.

MAHI MAHI

This zesty dish makes me feel like I'm on vacay on a beautiful island or dining at a fancy restaurant, which is crazy because it's so incredibly easy to make. Serve this with a crunchy salad and Food Babe's Favorite Green Beans on page 248.

Makes 4 servings
Prep Time: 5 minutes
Cook Time: 20 minutes
Total Time: 25 minutes

1 pound mahi mahi

1 tablespoon mayo (look for one with avocado oil)

2 teaspoons Dijon mustard

1 lemon, zested first, then juiced

½ teaspoon sea salt

¼ teaspoon paprika

Pinch of ground black pepper

1 lemon, sliced

Preheat the oven to 400°F. Place the mahi mahi in a baking dish.

In a small bowl, combine the mayo, mustard, lemon juice, zest, salt, paprika, and pepper.

Spread the mixture evenly on top of the mahi mahi. Add the sliced lemon on top and bake for 20 minutes.

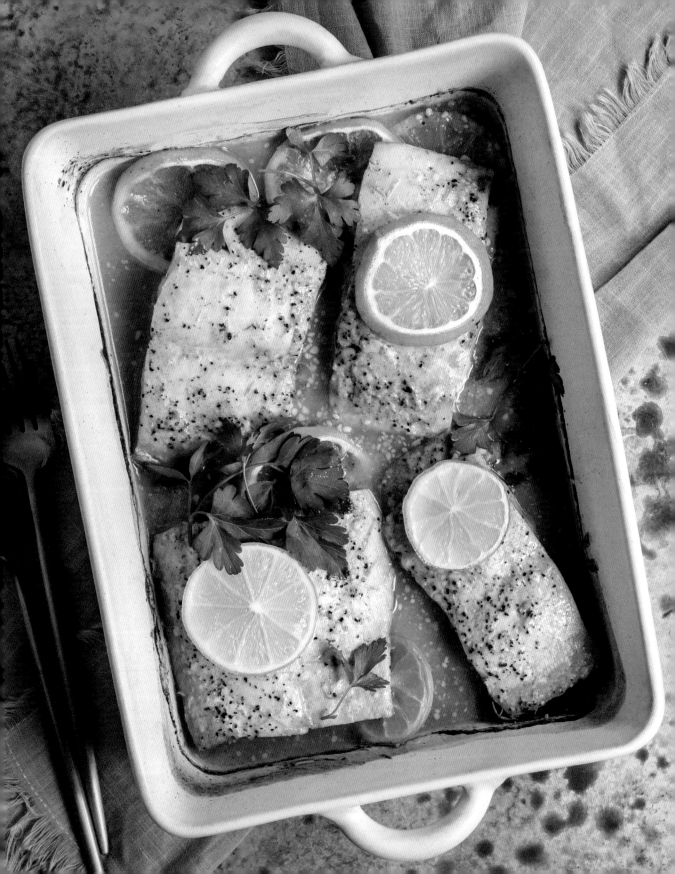

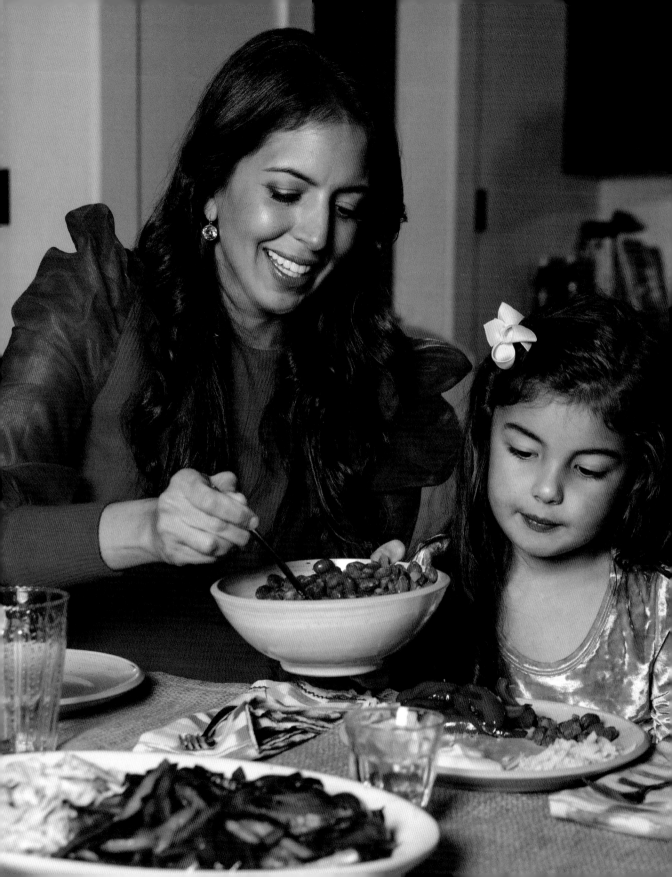

chapter 11

SIDES

COPYCAT "CHICK-FIL-A" WAFFLE FRIES

There's just something extra special about waffle fries. I don't know if it's the fun shape that makes them so delicious—but it certainly isn't all the processed ingredients that fast-food restaurants use to make theirs. I firmly believe that if you love to eat something, you can figure out how to make it at home with healthy ingredients. These fries are the perfect example of how to do this! Find the recipe for dipping sauces on page 211.

Makes 4 to 6 servings
Prep Time: 35 minutes
Cook Time: 30 minutes
Total Time: 65 minutes

3 medium-size Russet or Yukon Gold potatoes
2 to 3 tablespoons olive oil or coconut oil
1 teaspoon sea salt

Preheat the oven to 425°F.

Wash the potatoes and pat them dry. Using a mandolin on the thickest setting, slice the potatoes. Run each potato down across the blade to make the first slice. Turn the potato one quarter turn before making another slice. Continue this process until you have used the whole potato. Repeat with the remaining potatoes.

Place the slices in a bowl and fill it with cold water to ½ inch above the potatoes. Let them sit for 30 minutes.

Drain the water and dry the potatoes completely. A clean dish towel works well.

Toss the potatoes with the oil and salt, and spread them evenly on a parchment-lined baking sheet. Bake for 25 to 30 minutes or until golden brown. Turn the oven to broil and cook for 2 to 3 minutes to crisp the top, if needed. Let them cool slightly and serve immediately.

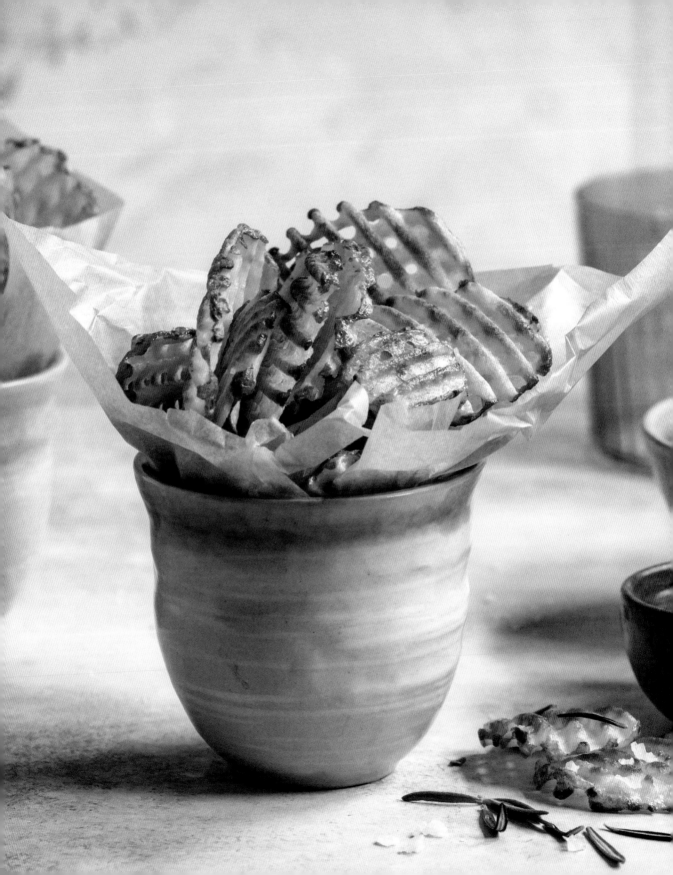

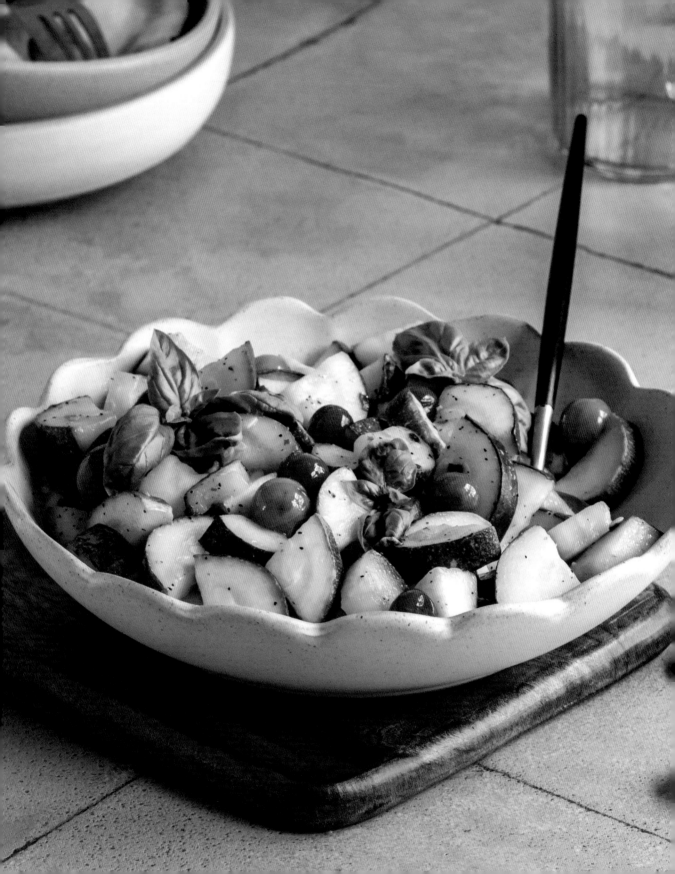

ZUCCHINI WITH SAUTÉED CHERRY TOMATOES

This fresh dish tastes like a garden of deliciousness. We love to use freshly plucked produce from our garden as much as possible, which is one reason why this recipe is in heavy rotation at our house. Serve this at your next summertime cookout with grilled chicken or fish.

Makes 4 servings
Prep Time: 5 minutes
Cook Time: 5 minutes
Total Time: 10 minutes

2 tablespoons olive oil
2 medium zucchinis, diced
1 cup cherry tomatoes
2 cloves garlic, minced
¼ teaspoon red pepper flakes
Sea salt, to taste
2 tablespoons chopped fresh basil

Heat the oil in a large skillet over medium-high heat.

Add the zucchini, cherry tomatoes, garlic, and red pepper flakes. Sauté until the zucchini is crisp-tender, about 5 minutes. Season with salt to taste.

Garnish with fresh chopped basil and serve.

FOOD BABE'S FAVORITE GREEN BEANS

My daughter loves to pick the pomegranate seeds out of this dish to eat them first! Which I'm totally okay with, since pomegranate seeds are a true superfood packed with antioxidants that help keep us healthy. This dish makes an amazing side during the holidays, since it looks so festive; but we love to serve these beans any day of the year.

Makes 4 servings
Prep Time: 7 minutes
Cook Time: 8 minutes
Total Time: 15 minutes

1 pound green beans, ends trimmed
1 to 2 tablespoons grass-fed butter
½ cup pomegranate seeds
Sea salt and ground black pepper, to taste

Bring a pot of water to boil and steam the green beans until desired doneness.

Transfer the cooked green beans to a bowl and mix in the butter and pomegranate seeds. Season with salt and pepper, as desired.

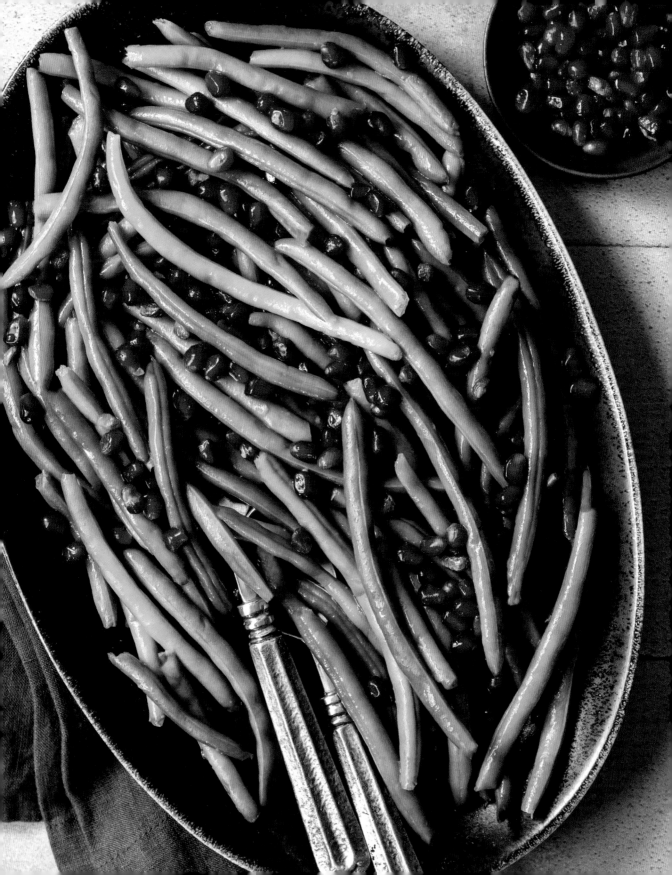

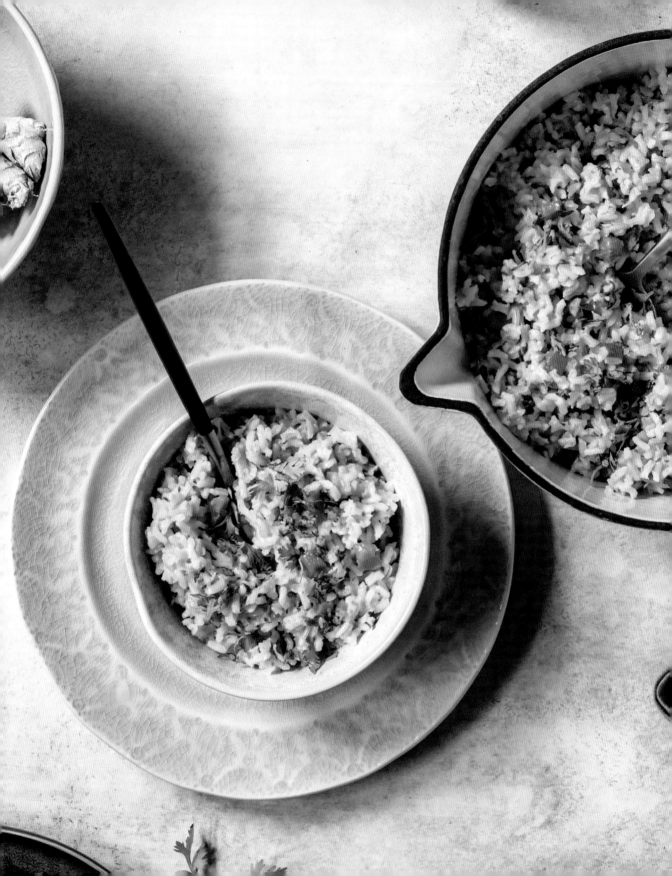

ONE-POT THAI-STYLE RICE

This quick "fried rice" cooks up in one pan. You can't beat the flavor of the fresh ginger root, cilantro, and turmeric simmered with the rice in coconut milk. It makes the perfect pairing to any stir-fry, but we love it with grilled chicken too.

Makes 4 to 6 servings
Prep Time: 10 minutes
Cook Time: 23 minutes
Total Time: 33 minutes

1 tablespoon coconut oil
¼ cup diced red onion
¼ cup diced carrots
1 cup brown basmati rice
1 cup coconut milk
¼ cup chopped fresh cilantro
1 teaspoon minced ginger root
¼ teaspoon ground turmeric
½ teaspoon sea salt
1 cup filtered water

Optional Toppings

1 lime, sliced
½ cup toasted cashews

Heat the oil in a pot over medium-high heat. Add the onion, carrots, and rice, and cook for 2 to 3 minutes.

Add the remaining ingredients along with the filtered water and bring to a boil. Reduce the heat and simmer the rice for 20 minutes or until the liquid has evaporated.

Stir in the toppings, if desired. Serve family style.

THE BEST SAUTÉED SPINACH

When you only have a few minutes to throw a side together, this is the ticket! This dish comes together with a splash of coconut aminos, which taste similar to soy sauce but with a touch of natural sweetness that makes the flavors in the spinach and onions pop. It pairs well with just about any main dish, so keep this one handy!

Makes 4 servings
Prep Time: 5 minutes
Cook Time: 3 minutes
Total Time: 8 minutes

1 tablespoon olive oil

½ small yellow onion, diced

3 garlic cloves, minced

8 ounces baby spinach (about 8 loose cups)

2 tablespoons coconut aminos

Squeeze of fresh lemon juice

Sea salt and freshly ground black pepper, to taste

Heat the olive oil in a large pot over medium-high heat. Add the onion and garlic and sauté for 2 minutes.

Add the spinach and coconut aminos and cook for about 1 minute, tossing the spinach with tongs occasionally until it is just wilted.

Take the pot off the heat and add a squeeze of lemon juice. Toss to combine and season with salt and pepper as needed. Serve immediately.

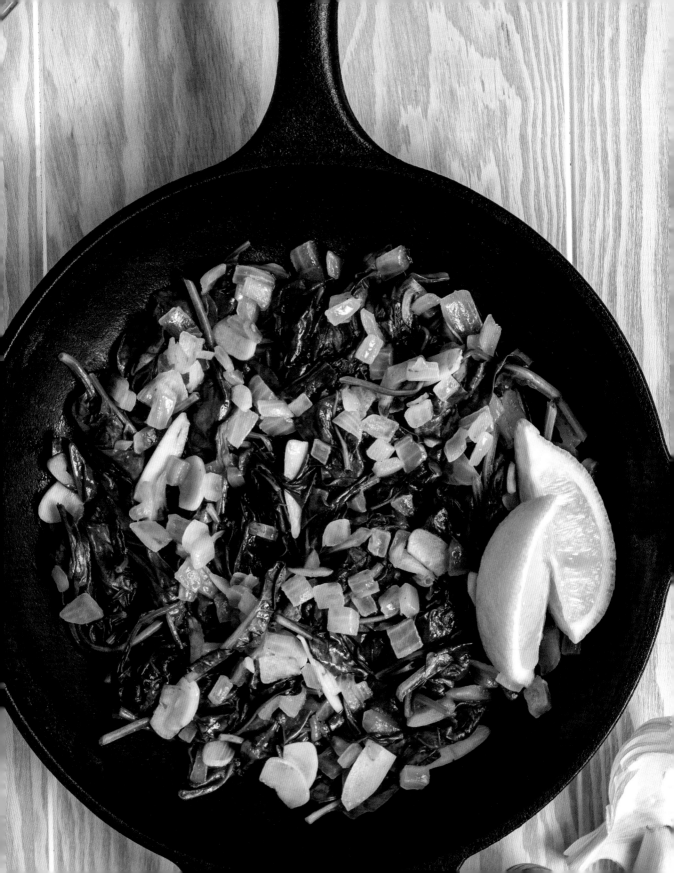

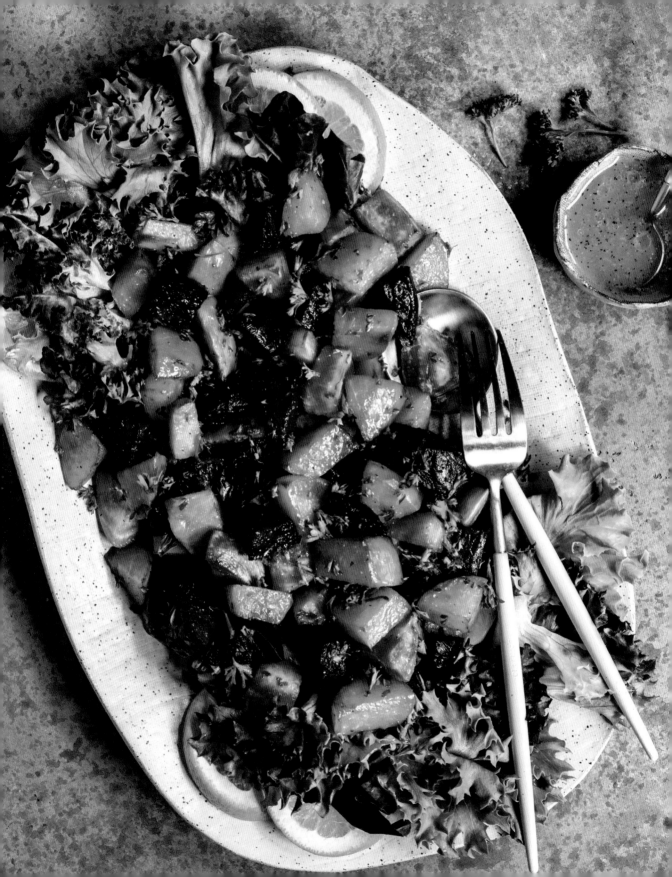

PERFECT MARINATED BEETS

I used to hate beets until I finally started preparing them myself. Those canned beets I was first exposed to in my school cafeteria totally scarred me until my late twenties. I'm so happy to love them now—they are incredible vegetables that help cleanse the blood. And who doesn't need a little cleansing after all the nasty stuff we are exposed to day in and day out?

Makes 4 servings
Prep Time: 10 minutes
Cook Time: 30 to 35 minutes
Total Time: 40 minutes

6 to 8 medium beets, tops trimmed, peeled and diced
1 to 2 tablespoons olive oil
½ teaspoon sea salt
¼ teaspoon ground black pepper
½ orange, juiced
2 tablespoons red wine vinegar
¼ cup chopped fresh parsley

Preheat the oven to 375°F.

Place the beets in a baking dish and drizzle them with olive oil, salt, and pepper. Bake for 30 to 35 minutes or until they are fork tender.

In a small bowl, mix together the orange juice and vinegar. Pour the mixture over the beets and toss to combine. Garnish with fresh parsley and serve immediately.

EASY PARMESAN BROCCOLI

I eat cruciferous veggies like broccoli often because they are superstars in the vegetable family. They can help remove toxins from the body by boosting the liver's own detoxifying enzymes. There is research out there that shows cruciferous veggies may help to stave off cancer and heart disease too. So, if you're not doing so already, it's time to add broccoli (and other cruciferous veggies like kale and cauliflower) to your diet STAT. This broccoli dish is great with grilled chicken, fish, or pasta.

Makes 4 servings
Prep Time: 5 minutes
Cook Time: 4 minutes
Total Time: 9 minutes

1 large head broccoli, cut into florets (reserve the stems for another use)

1 to 2 tablespoons grass-fed butter

½ lemon, juiced

¼ cup freshly grated Parmesan cheese

Sea salt and ground black pepper, to taste

Steam the broccoli to desired doneness, about 4 minutes for crisp-tender.

Drain the broccoli. Add the butter and lemon juice to the pot and melt the butter. Return the broccoli to the pot and toss to coat it with the melted butter. Add the Parmesan and toss again. Season with salt and pepper and serve.

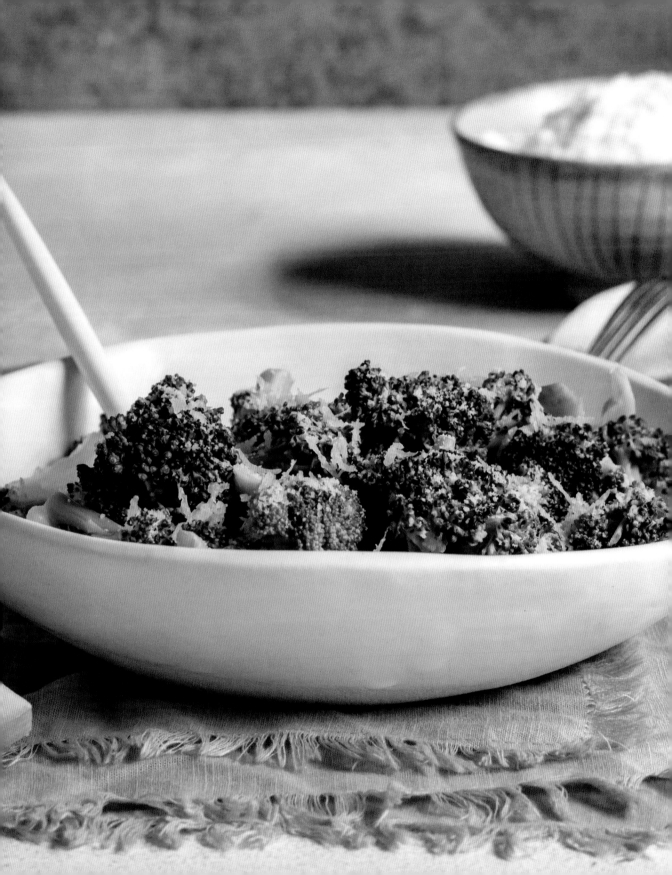

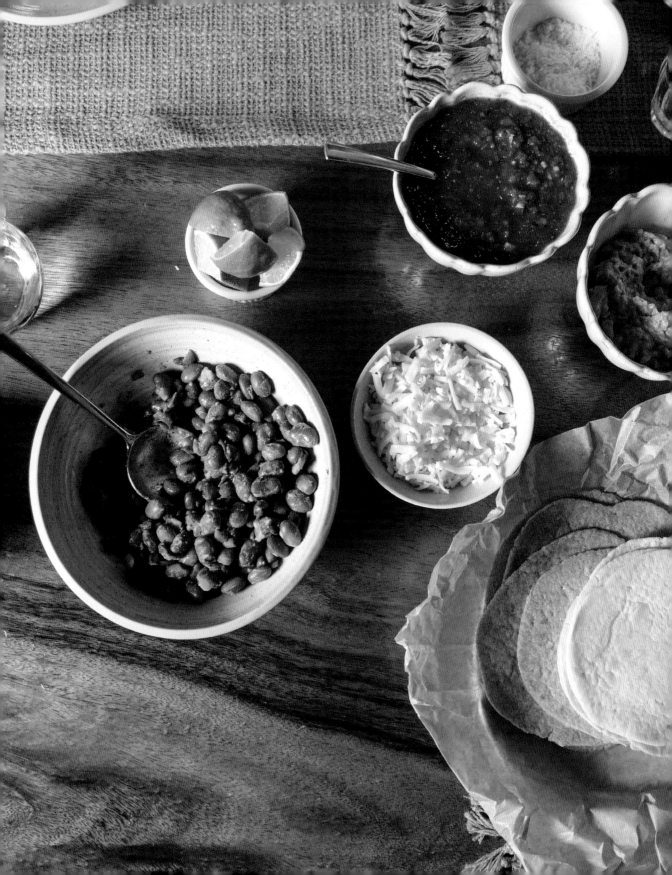

PINTO BEANS

This is the must-have taco night accompaniment. I also love to serve these beans with Mexican-style rice or tortillas for a quick, meatless meal. Add some sliced avocado, sour cream, or cheese. These beans are great for fajita night, to freeze in small portions for lunches, or to add to burritos.

Makes 4 servings
Prep Time: 5 minutes
Cook Time: 8 hours
Total Time: 8 hours 5 minutes

2 cups dried pinto beans, soaked overnight

1 yellow onion, skin removed and cut in half

3 garlic cloves, peeled

1 jalapeño, seeded and diced

2 teaspoons sea salt

½ teaspoon ground cumin

Drain the soaked beans and place them in a slow cooker. Cover the beans with 1 inch of water.

Add the onion, garlic, jalapeño, salt, and cumin. Stir to combine. Cook on low for 8 hours.

ROASTED CAULIFLOWER

When I was a kid, I wasn't a big fan of cauliflower. Looking back, I think I just didn't have enough courage to try different dishes. Now I really love it, especially when it is roasted. Preparing cauliflower this way makes it so flavorful and only takes a few minutes of prep work in the kitchen. If you think you or your children don't like cauliflower, give this one a try. It might surprise you!

Makes 4 servings
Prep Time: 5 minutes
Cook Time: 30 minutes
Total Time: 35 minutes

1 head cauliflower, cut into florets
2 tablespoons olive oil
1 teaspoon paprika
½ teaspoon sea salt
¼ teaspoon ground black pepper

Preheat the oven to 375°F.

Place the florets on a parchment-lined baking sheet. Toss with the olive oil, paprika, salt, and pepper. Bake for 30 minutes.

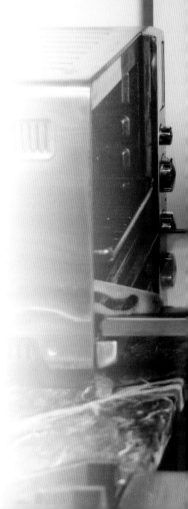

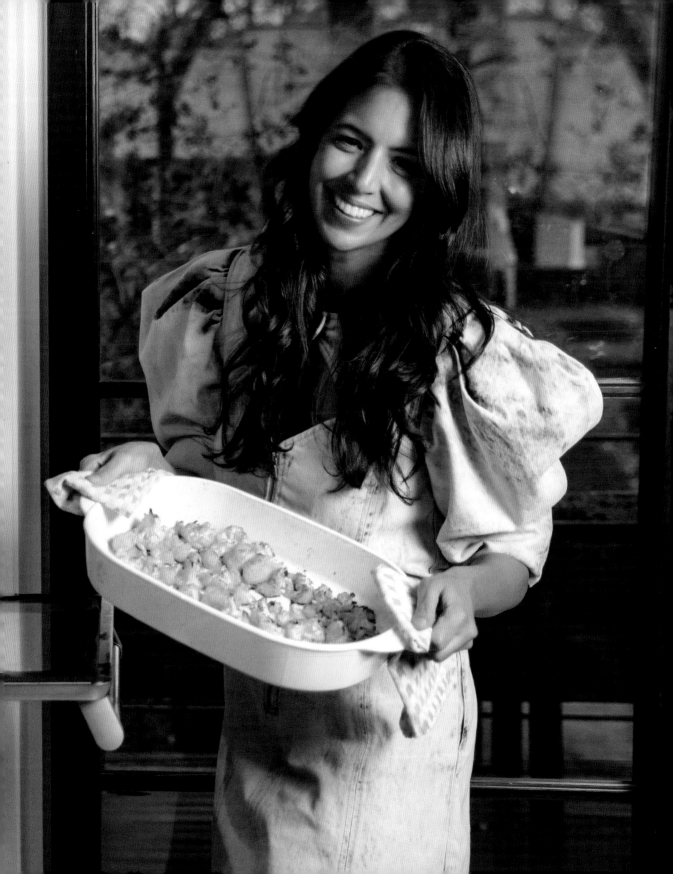

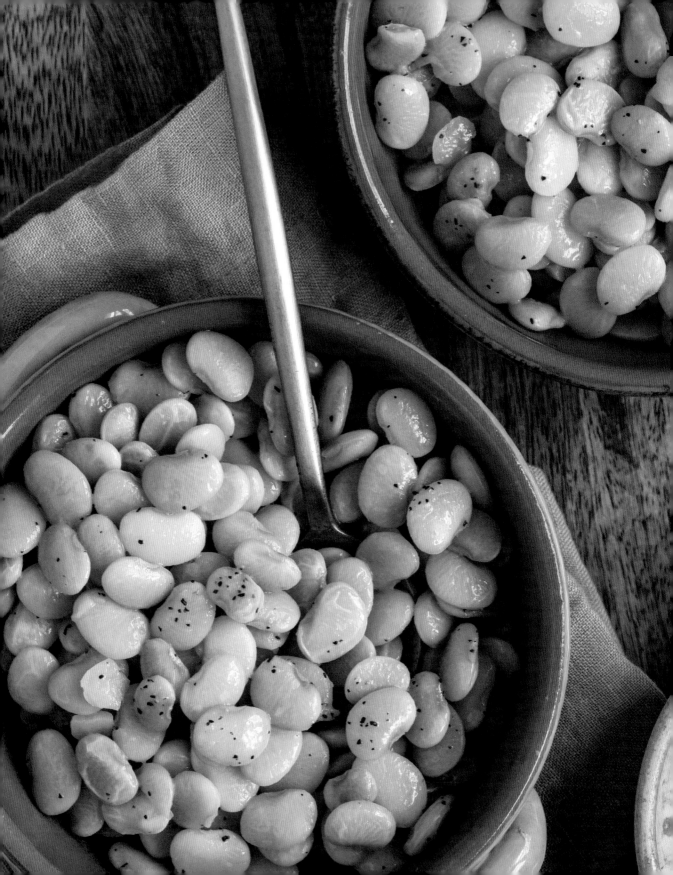

BUTTER BEANS

Stop turning the page and bookmark this recipe. I know, I know . . . you may have hated lima beans as a child, but trust me on this one. Preparing these beans simply with butter, salt, and pepper is the way to go. My entire family gobbles these up!

Makes 4 servings
Prep Time: 5 minutes
Cook Time: 20 minutes
Total Time: 25 minutes

2 cups frozen lima beans
½ teaspoon sea salt
2 tablespoons grass-fed butter
Ground black pepper, to taste

Place the lima beans and salt in a pot and add enough water to cover them. Bring to a boil and cook the beans for 15 to 20 minutes.

Drain the beans and toss them with the butter, pepper, and additional salt, if needed.

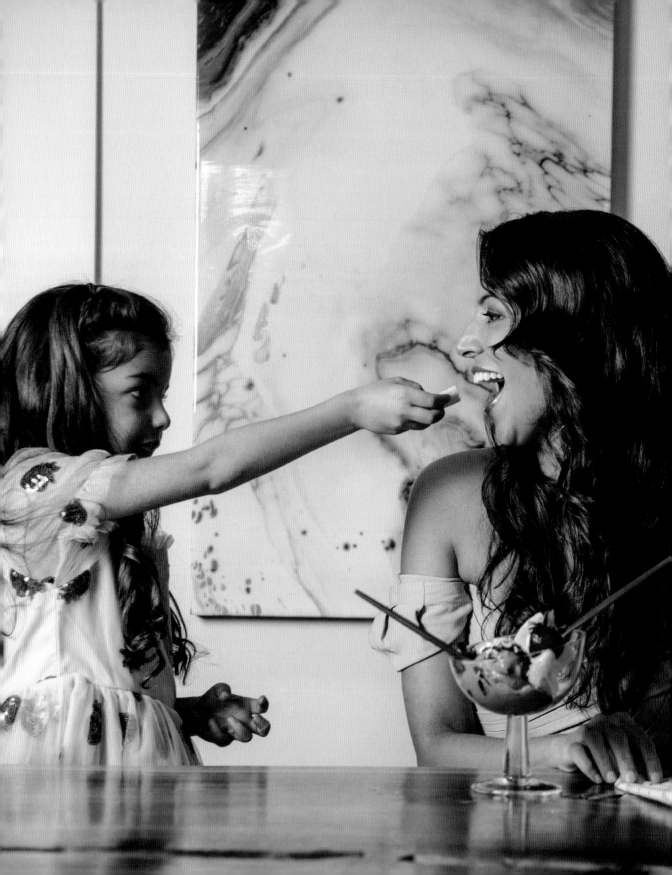

chapter 12

DESSERTS

BAREFOOT IN THE PARK COOKIES

This is my favorite organic vegan cookie. It's amazing that you don't need any butter, oil, or eggs to make an awesome little cookie! I call them Barefoot in the Park cookies because I was inspired to make these oatmeal-raisin treats after a fun day in the park with my girlfriends.

Makes 10 to 12 cookies
Prep Time: 10 minutes
Cook Time: 15 minutes
Total Time: 25 minutes

1 cup whole wheat pastry flour or spelt flour
1 cup rolled oats
1 cup unsweetened coconut flakes
½ cup raisins
⅓ cup coconut sugar
1 teaspoon ground cinnamon
½ teaspoon baking soda
½ teaspoon ground cardamom
¼ teaspoon sea salt
½ cup unsweetened applesauce
¼ cup pure maple syrup
1 teaspoon vanilla extract

Preheat the oven to 350°F.

In a bowl, mix together all the dry ingredients.

In a separate bowl, combine the applesauce, maple syrup, and vanilla.

Slowly add the dry ingredients to the wet and mix until combined.

Shape the dough into balls using a level ⅓ cup of dough for each cookie. Place the dough balls on heavy large parchment-lined baking sheets, spacing them apart. Gently flatten the dough with your fingertips into 3 ½-inch rounds. (Dip your fingers in water to prevent the dough from sticking to them.)

Bake the cookies until they are golden brown, about 15 minutes. Let them cool on a wire rack before serving. You can store these cookies in an airtight container for up to 4 days.

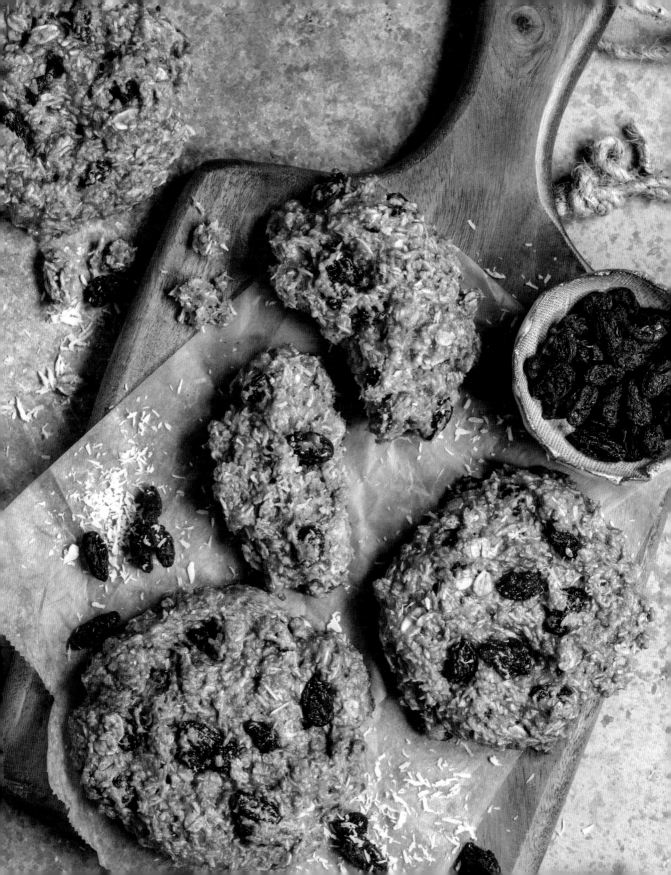

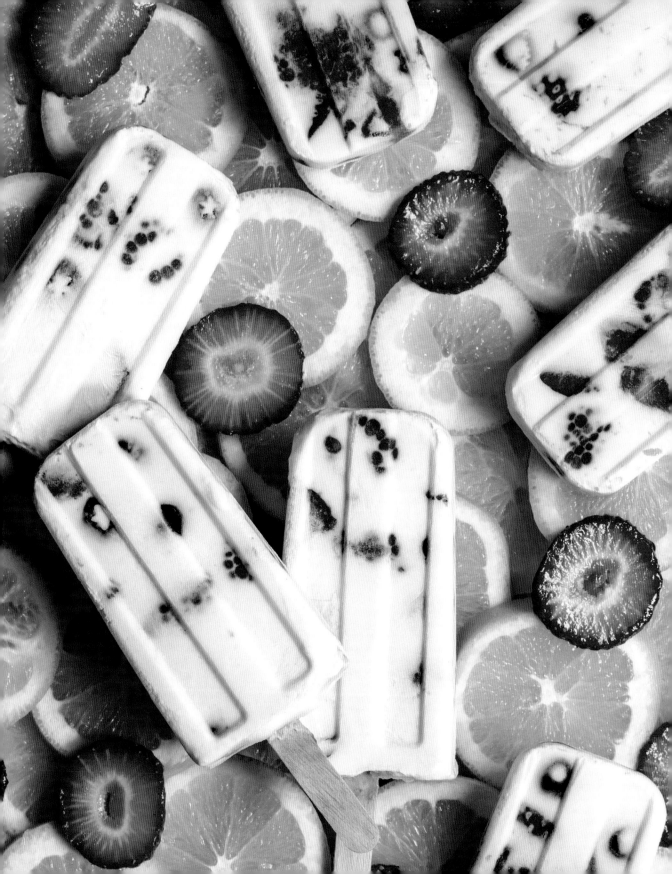

COCONUT CREAMSICLE BERRY POPS

Store-bought frozen treats and ice cream bars are usually made with refined and processed sugars, gut-destroying emulsifiers like carrageenan and cellulose gum, GMOs, and all sorts of other ingredients that no one should have to consume to enjoy a treat! This is why I love making these Coconut Creamsicle Berry Pops. They are dairy free and absolutely deeeeeelicious!

Makes 5 to 8 servings (number of servings depends on size of popsicle molds)
Prep Time: 5 minutes, plus at least 6 hours to freeze

1¼ cups canned coconut milk

1 large orange, juiced (about ⅓ cup juice)

1½ teaspoons finely grated orange zest

2 tablespoons pure maple syrup or raw honey

Heaping ½ cup mixed berries (if using strawberries, you might want to dice them into smaller pieces)

Place all the ingredients into a large pitcher or bowl and mix well.

Fill popsicle molds to the top and place the popsicle stick in the mold.

Place the molds in the freezer until the popsicles are fully frozen, at least 6 hours or overnight.

Dip the molds in a bowl of hot water to loosen them.

SUPERFOOD POPS

Don't waste your money on boxes full of processed chemicals, because it's super easy to make frozen treats with healthy ingredients—even SUPERFOODS! All you need are a few good healthy ingredients to make these Superfood Pops, which pack a super nutritional punch in each bite.

Makes 4 to 6 servings
Prep Time: 5 minutes, plus at least 2 hours to freeze

PINEAPPLE GINGER POPS

1 cup chopped pineapple

1 teaspoon grated ginger root, plus more as desired

¼ teaspoon ground turmeric

½ cup coconut milk

2 teaspoons raw honey

Place all of the ingredients in a blender and blend well.

Pour the mixture into popsicle molds and place them in the freezer for at least 2 hours (or overnight).

SWEET GREEN POPS

1 apple, cored

2 cups kale

1 cucumber

½ lemon, juiced

Wash the apple and vegetables thoroughly and dry.

Place all the ingredients in a juicer, except the lemon juice. Add the lemon juice to the juice container and stir to combine. If you do not have a juicer, you can use a blender and strain the liquid through a fine mesh strainer or cheesecloth.

Pour the mixture into popsicle molds and place them in the freezer for at least 2 hours (or overnight).

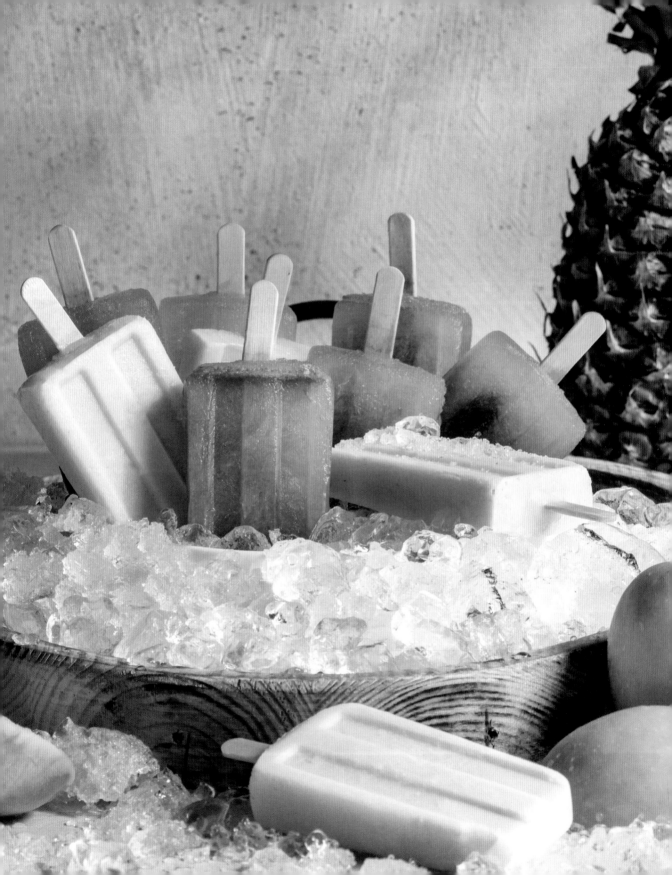

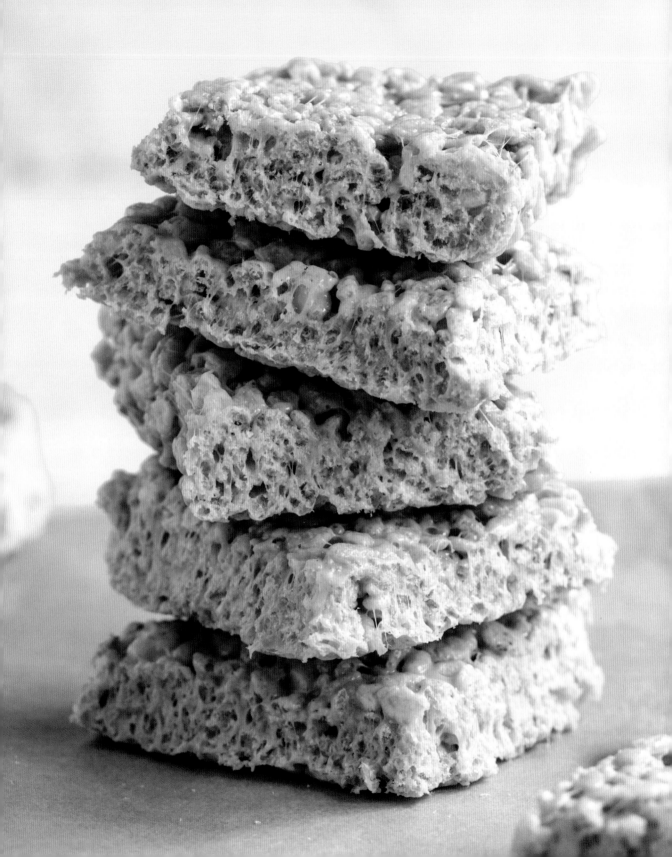

BETTER-FOR-YOU "RICE KRISPIES" TREATS

DISCLAIMER: I can polish off half of a pan of these "Rice Krispies" Treats in one sitting, so if you make these, don't get mad at me—you've been warned. I grew up with homemade treats similar to these, but the ingredients were totally different. Did you know they add artificial blue dye to most marshmallows to make them look brighter? Yikes! Nowadays, I make these treats with brown rice crispy cereal and the best natural marshmallows I can find without dyes.

Makes 9 to 12 squares
Prep Time: 10 minutes

3 tablespoons grass-fed butter

4 ½ ounces natural marshmallows
(about 2 ¾ cups)
(I use Hammond's Vanilla Bean Marshmallows.)

6 cups brown rice crisps

Melt the 3 tablespoons of butter in a saucepan over medium heat.

Add the marshmallows and heat them until they are melted, stirring as needed. Take the saucepan off the stove.

Stir in the brown rice crisps and mix until everything is well combined. Press the mixture into a buttered baking pan. Allow the treats to cool fully before cutting them into squares.

5-MINUTE CHOCOLATE PUDDING CUPS

Not only is this chocolate pudding lightning-quick to make, but it's sweetened with a touch of pure maple syrup and the natural sweetness found in coconut and vanilla. When you top it with some high-fiber berries, such as raspberries or blackberries, you'll help to slow the absorption of those natural sugars in the body, which is much healthier than eating traditional, sugar-loaded pudding cups. (And these are actually more delicious than those chemical-filled cups anyway.)

Makes 4 to 6 servings
Prep Time: 5 minutes

2 cups coconut cream
¼ cup canned coconut milk
¼ cup cacao powder
¼ cup pure maple syrup
2 teaspoons vanilla extract
½ teaspoon ground cinnamon
Pinch of sea salt

Optional Toppings

Fresh berries

Cacao nibs

Place all the ingredients in a blender and blend on high until smooth and creamy. Pour into a bowl, cover, and place in the refrigerator for at least 1 hour to set.

Add ½ cup of pudding to a glass dessert cup and serve with fresh berries or cacao nibs.

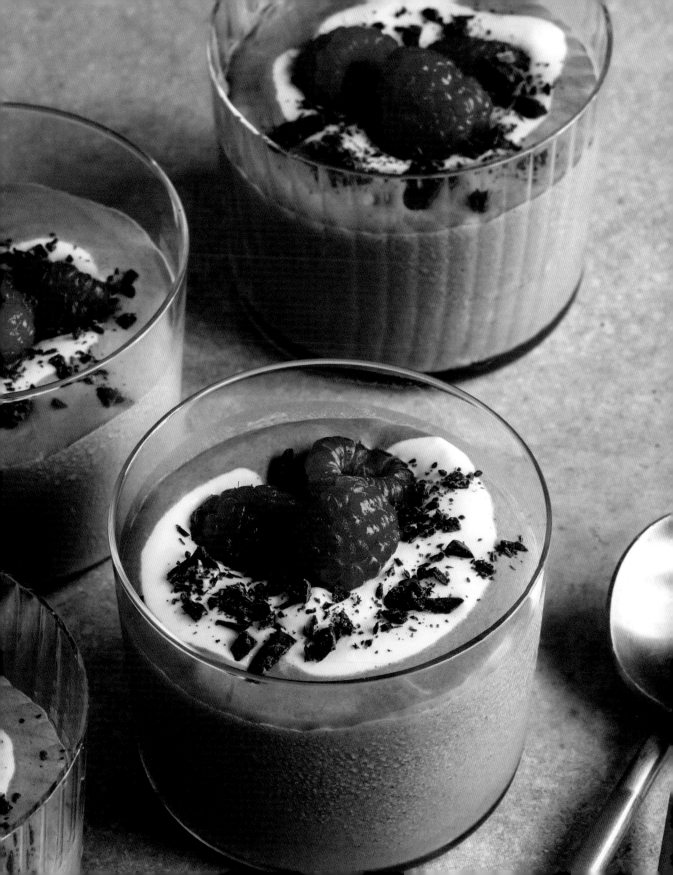

HOMEMADE "OREOS"

Pretty much nothing gets my family more excited than baking a batch of these super-stuffed "Oreos." Dunking these bad boys in milk brings me back to my childhood, and I love knowing that the ingredients are stellar compared to the store-bought version. My kids love to help spread the filling and can't wait to take a bite. Pop one open and lick the frosting out first. You can thank me later!

Makes 18 to 20 cookies
Prep Time: 20 minutes
Cook Time: 12 minutes
Total Time: 32 minutes

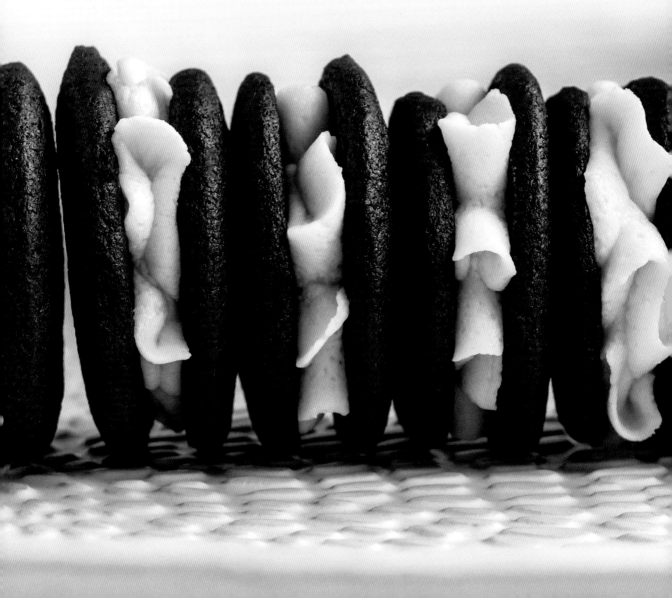

1 ½ cups spelt flour
(gluten-free: use oat flour)

½ cup unsweetened dark cocoa powder

1 teaspoon baking soda

½ teaspoon sea salt

½ cup butter, softened

1 cup coconut sugar

1 egg

2 teaspoons vanilla extract

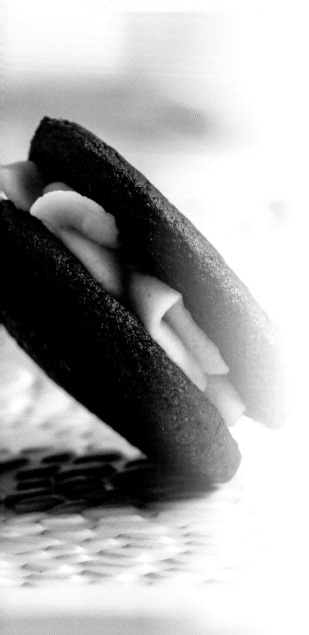

CREAM FILLING

4 tablespoons butter, softened

¼ cup cream cheese

1 cup powdered sugar

1 teaspoon vanilla extract

Preheat the oven to 350°F.

In a bowl, mix the flour, cocoa powder, baking soda, and salt. Set aside.

In a separate bowl, beat the butter and sugar together until smooth, about 1 to 2 minutes. Add the egg and vanilla and beat until combined.

Slowly add the dry ingredients to the wet. Mix until the batter forms a ball and begins to pull away from the sides.

Roll out the dough between two sheets of parchment paper until it is roughly ¼ inch thick.

Use a small round cookie cutter to cut shapes out of the dough. Place the shapes on a parchment-lined baking sheet and bake for 10 to 12 minutes. Let cool.

While the cookies are baking, make the cream filling. Place all the ingredients in a bowl and beat until light and fluffy.

To assemble, take one of the cookies and spread roughly 1 tablespoon of cream filling on top. Add another cookie on top and enjoy!

COPYCAT TOASTER STRUDEL

These flaky and buttery pastries are deadly delicious. And even better, they are ridiculously easy to make though they look so fancy. You'll impress your family and friends with your mad cooking skills. Don't worry, I won't tell anyone that you didn't spend hours in the kitchen making these. It's our little secret.

Makes 4 servings
Prep Time: 10 minutes
Cook Time: 20 minutes
Total Time: 30 minutes

½ cup jam of choice (see homemade jams recipe on page 163)

½ tablespoon arrowroot powder

1 egg

1 tablespoon heavy cream

One 14-ounce package of puff pastry, thawed

ICING

½ cup powdered sugar

½ teaspoon vanilla extract

Drop of almond extract (optional)

2 to 3 tablespoons heavy cream, more as needed

Preheat the oven to 400°F. Line a baking sheet with parchment paper and set it aside.

In a small bowl, mix together the jam and arrowroot powder. Set aside.

In a separate bowl, whisk together the egg and heavy cream.

Cut the sheet of puff pastry into 8 equal rectangles. Spoon 1 heaping tablespoon of jam onto the center of 4 rectangles, leaving roughly ½ inch of pastry around the edges.

Lightly brush the edges of one of the rectangles with the egg wash. Place a jam-free puff pastry rectangle on top and seal the edges using the back of a fork. Place the assembled strudel on the prepared baking sheet. Repeat the process with the remaining ingredients.

Brush the tops of each strudel with the egg wash. Bake them for 20 to 22 minutes or until they are golden brown. Let them cool a bit.

While the strudels are baking, make the icing by mixing all the ingredients in a bowl; add more cream if the mixture is too thick. Once the strudels have cooled, drizzle the icing on top and serve.

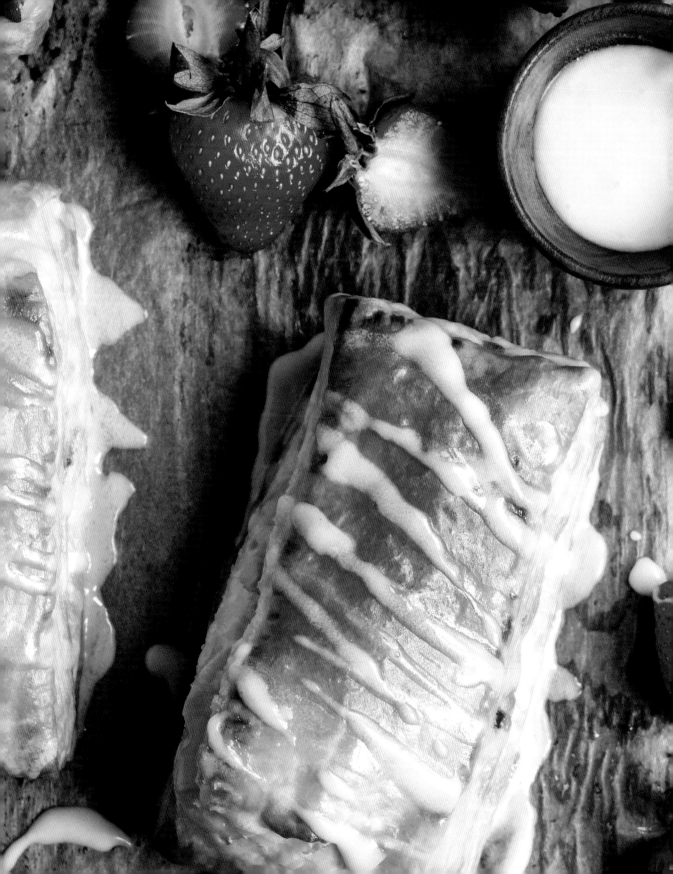

OATMEAL CREAM PIE COOKIES

If you tried to read the ingredient list on a box of Little Debbie Oatmeal Creme Pies you'd probably die from exhaustion before reaching the end. The list is a mile long, with so many man-made additives that it will make your head spin. This makes me incredibly sad knowing how many children eat these snacks. That's why I created this homemade alternative, which is really fun to bake with your children and include as a special treat in their lunch box.

Makes 8 sandwich cookies
Prep Time: 35 minutes
Cook Time: 12 minutes
Total Time: 47 minutes

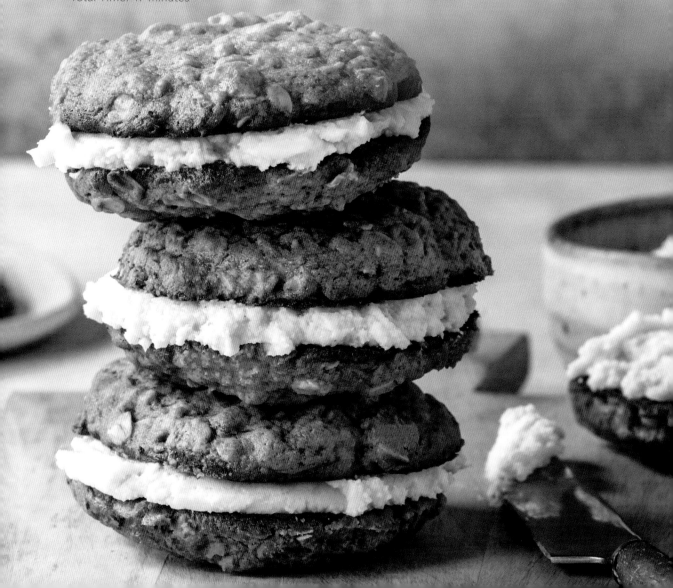

½ cup grass-fed butter, softened

1 cup coconut sugar

1 egg

1 tablespoon molasses

1 teaspoon vanilla extract

1 cup spelt or oat flour

1 cup rolled oats

1 teaspoon baking powder

½ teaspoon ground cinnamon

½ teaspoon sea salt

Preheat the oven to 350°F.

To make the cookies: Cream the butter and sugar together in a bowl until the mixture is light and fluffy, about 1 to 2 minutes. Add the egg, molasses, and vanilla and mix to combine.

In a separate bowl, mix the flour, oats, baking powder, cinnamon, and salt. Add this to the butter mixture and stir until just combined.

Use a scant 2 tablespoons of dough for each cookie. Drop the dough onto heavy large parchment-lined baking sheets, spacing each cookie roughly 2 inches apart (about 8 cookies per sheet). Using wet fingertips, flatten them into 2-inch rounds. Bake the cookies until they are golden brown, about 12 minutes. Let them cool completely.

BUTTERCREAM FILLING

½ cup butter, softened

1 ½ cups powdered sugar

1 to 2 tablespoons milk of choice

1 teaspoon vanilla extract

To make the buttercream filling: Combine the ingredients in a bowl and beat them until the mixture is light and fluffy.

When the cookies have completely cooled, spread 1½ to 2 tablespoons of buttercream evenly onto the flat side of half of them. Top each with another cookie. Refrigerate in an airtight container for up to 3 days.

CLASSIC APPLE PIE

When I realized the pies in supermarket bakeries were filled with corn syrup, chemical preservatives, and refined oils (instead of real butter), I decided it was time to make my own. And boy am I glad that I did! This homemade apple pie blows those processed pies away. You'll love how delicious it makes your house smell while it's baking too. You'll want to make this pie every year for the holidays and any time your family is cozying up at home on a cold day.

Makes 8 servings
Prep Time: 1 hour
Cook Time: 1 hour 12 minutes
Total Time: 2 hours 12 minutes

PIE CRUST

2 ½ cups organic unbleached all-purpose flour

2 teaspoons coconut sugar

¼ teaspoon sea salt

½ cup (1 stick) chilled grass-fed butter, diced

FILLING

4 Granny Smith apples (1 pound 11 ounces), peeled and cut into ¼-inch-thick slices

3 assorted apples of choice (1 pound 6 ounces), peeled and cut into ¼-inch-thick slices (Honeycrisp, Golden Delicious or Braeburn work well)

½ cup (1 stick) grass-fed butter

¼ cup organic unbleached all-purpose flour

¼ cup filtered water

1 cup coconut sugar

2 tablespoons fresh lemon juice

1 teaspoon ground cinnamon

1 egg, beaten (for brushing on top)

To make the pie crust: Place the flour, sugar, and salt in a food processor. Pulse to combine. Add the butter and pulse until crumbs form. Add 11 tablespoons of ice water and pulse until the dough just starts to come together, adding more water by tablespoonfuls if necessary.

Gather the dough into a ball. Divide the dough in half, and flatten each half into a disk. Wrap the disks in a clean kitchen towel and refrigerate them for 1 hour.

To make the filling: Slice the apples and place the slices in a large bowl; set aside.

Melt the butter in a heavy saucepan over medium heat. Add the flour and whisk for roughly 1 minute. Add the filtered water, whisking constantly until combined. Add the sugar, lemon juice, and cinnamon and whisk for 30 seconds.

Pour the mixture over the apples and mix well to combine.

Position the rack in the lower third of the oven and preheat the oven to 350°F.

Roll out 1 dough disk between sheets of parchment paper to a 12-inch round (the dough will be thin). Carefully peel off the

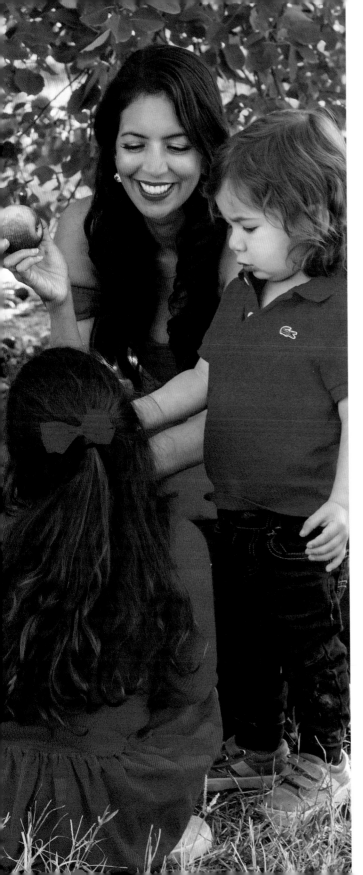

top sheet of parchment. Invert the dough into a 9-inch pie dish; carefully peel off the other piece of parchment. Gently press the dough into the dish.

Mound the apple filling in the dough-lined dish.

Roll out the second dough disk between layers of parchment paper into a 12-inch round. Peel off the top sheet of parchment. Invert the dough over the filling; carefully remove the other piece of parchment. Crimp the top and bottom dough edges together to seal the pie. Make 5 evenly spaced slits in the top of the pie. Brush the top of the pie with the beaten egg.

Bake the pie until the apples are tender when pierced with a sharp knife, filling bubbles thickly, and the crust is golden brown, about 1 hour 10 minutes (cover loosely with foil if the top is becoming too brown). Cool the pie for at least 1 hour before serving.

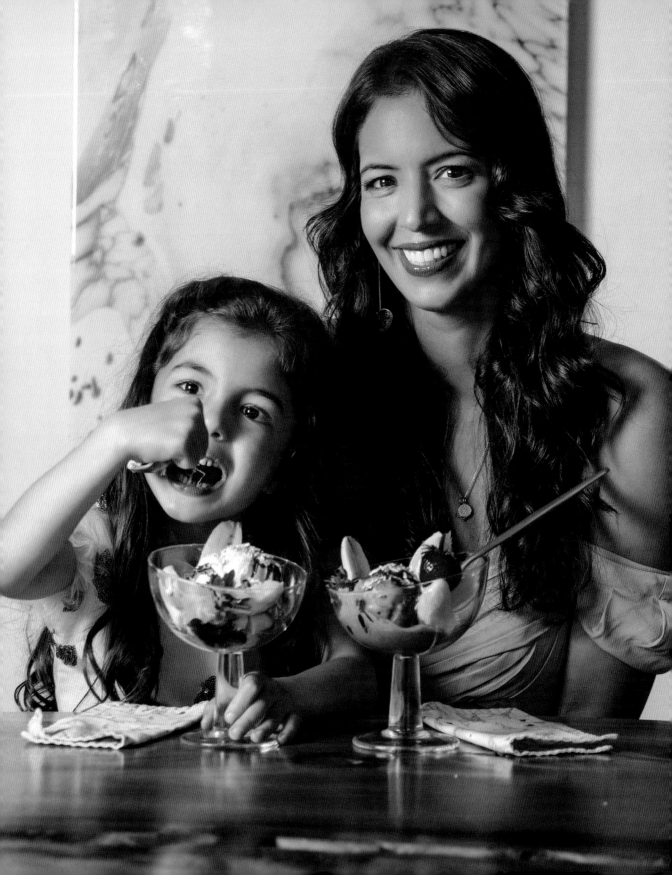

BANANA SPLIT

This decadent dessert is a showstopper. Just thinking about these banana splits makes me drool. We create our own "hot fudge" with organic chocolate (we like Hu Gems) and coconut oil, which we drizzle over bananas and organic store-bought ice cream (such as Cosmic Bliss). Everyone gets their choice of fun toppings like strawberries, cacao nibs, and whipped cream before digging in!

Makes 1 serving
Prep Time: 5 minutes
Cook Time: 5 minutes
Total Time: 10 minutes

BANANA SPLIT

½ cup dark chocolate
1 tablespoon coconut oil
1 ripe banana, peeled and cut lengthwise
3 scoops ice cream of your choice
Handful fresh strawberries, chopped
¼ cup chopped nuts of choice (optional)
1 to 2 tablespoons cacao nibs (optional)
3 fresh cherries

To make the hot fudge topping: Melt the chocolate and coconut oil in a double boiler, stirring as needed. Set aside.

To assemble the banana split: Place the banana slices on a plate or long, shallow dish. Top them with 3 scoops of ice cream.

Drizzle the chocolate mix over the ice cream and bananas. Add the chopped fresh strawberries and nuts and/or cacao nibs if using. Finish the banana split with a dollop or two of whipped cream and the fresh cherries.

FRESH WHIPPED CREAM

1 pint heavy whipping cream (16 ounces)
1 tablespoon of vanilla extract
3 tablespoons of organic powdered sugar

To make the fresh whipped cream: Whip the heavy cream, vanilla, and sugar in a large mixing bowl until creamy and smooth.

METRIC CONVERSION CHART

Standard Cup	Fine Powder (e.g., flour)	Grain (e.g., rice)	Granular (e.g., sugar)	Liquid Solids (e.g., butter)	Liquid (e.g., milk)
1	140 g	150 g	190 g	200 g	240 ml
¾	105 g	113 g	143 g	150 g	180 ml
⅔	93 g	100 g	125 g	133 g	160 ml
½	70 g	75 g	95 g	100 g	120 ml
⅓	47 g	50 g	63 g	67 g	80 ml
¼	35 g	38 g	48 g	50 g	60 ml
⅛	18 g	19 g	24 g	25 g	30 ml

Useful Equivalents for Cooking/Oven Temperatures

Process	Fahrenheit	Celsius	Gas Mark
Freeze Water	32° F	0° C	
Room Temperature	68° F	20° C	
Boil Water	212° F	100° C	
Bake	325° F	160° C	3
	350° F	180° C	4
	375° F	190° C	5
	400° F	200° C	6
	425° F	220° C	7
	450° F	230° C	8
Broil			Grill

Useful Equivalents for Liquid Ingredients by Volume

¼ tsp			1 ml
½ tsp			2 ml
1 tsp			5 ml
3 tsp	1 tbsp	½ fl oz	15 ml
	2 tbsp	⅛ cup	1 fl oz	30 ml
	4 tbsp	¼ cup	2 fl oz	60 ml
	5⅓ tbsp	⅓ cup	3 fl oz	80 ml
	8 tbsp	½ cup	4 fl oz	120 ml
	10⅔ tbsp	⅔ cup	5 fl oz	160 ml
	12 tbsp	¾ cup	6 fl oz	180 ml
	16 tbsp	1 cup	8 fl oz	240 ml
	1 pt	2 cups	16 fl oz	480 ml
	1 qt	4 cups	32 fl oz	960 ml

Useful Equivalents for Dry Ingredients by Weight

(To convert ounces to grams, multiply the number of ounces by 30.)

1 oz	1/16 lb	30 g
4 oz	¼ lb	120 g
8 oz	½ lb	240 g
12 oz	¾ lb	360 g
16 oz	1 lb	480 g

Useful Equivalents for Length

(To convert inches to centimeters, multiply the number of inches by 2.5.)

1 in			2.5 cm
6 in	½ ft		15 cm
12 in	1 ft		30 cm
36 in	3 ft	1 yd	90 cm
40 in			100 cm	1 m

ENDNOTES

Introduction

1. Adekunle Sanyaolu, et al., "Childhood and Adolescent Obesity in the United States: A Public Health Concern," *Global Pediatric Health*, 6, no. 2333794X19891305 (December 1, 2019). https://www.ncbi.nlm.nih.gov/pmc /articles/PMC6887808. "Rates of New Diagnosed Cases of Type 1 and Type 2 Diabetes Continue to Rise Among Children, Teens," Centers for Disease Control and Prevention, accessed November 4, 2022, https:// www.cdc.gov/diabetes/research/reports/children-diabetes-rates-rise.html. "Key Statistics for Childhood Cancers," American Cancer Society, accessed November 4, 2022, https://www.cancer .org/cancer/cancer-in-children/key-statistics.html.

Chapter 1

1. "Picky Eaters," UCSF Benioff Children's Hospitals, accessed November 4, 2022, https://www. ucsfbenioffchildrens.org/education/picky-eaters.

2. "In Baby's 'First Bite,' A Chance to Shape a Child's Taste," *Fresh Air*, NPR, February 4, 2016, https://www.npr .org/sections/thesalt/2016/02/04/465305656/in-babys-first-bite-a-chance-to-shape-a-childs-taste.

3. University of Colorado Anschutz Medical Campus, "Lack of Vegetable Choices in Infant and Toddler Food Is Widespread," *ScienceDaily*, accessed November 4, 2022, www.sciencedaily.com/releases/2018/04 /180410110855.htm.

4. "Is It Safe for Babies to Eat Eggs?" *Healthline*, accessed November 4, 2022, https://www.healthline.com /health/parenting/when-can-a-baby-eat-eggs.

5. Jennifer Koplin, et al., "Can Early Introduction of Egg Prevent Egg Allergy in Infants? A Population-based Study," *Journal of Allergy and Clinical Immunology*, 126, no. 4 (October 2010): 807. https://www.jacionline .org/article/S0091-6749(10)01173-5/fulltext.

6. "Heavy Metals in Baby Food: What You Need to Know," *Consumer Reports*, last modified September 29, 2021, https://www.consumerreports.org/food-safety/heavy-metals-in-baby-food-a6772370847.

7. "Consumer Reports Calls on Baby Food Companies to Suspend Sales of Infant Rice Cereals, Citing Recent Government Test Results and Recalls," *Advocacy*, Consumer Reports, October 20, 2021, https://advocacy .consumerreports.org/press_release/infantricecereal10202021.

8. "Beech-Nut Nutrition Company Issues a Voluntary Recall of One Lot of Beech-Nut Single Grain Rice Cereal and Also Decides to Exit the Rice Cereal Segment," U.S. Food & Drug Administration, last modified June 8, 2021, https://www.fda.gov/safety/recalls-market-withdrawals-safety-alerts/beech-nut-nutrition-company-issues-voluntary-recall-one-lot-beech-nut-single-grain-rice-cereal-and.

9. Kevin Loria, "Why You Should Consider Alternatives to Infant Rice Cereal," *Consumer Reports*, last modified February 17, 2022, https://www.consumerreports.org/baby-food/why-you-should-consider-alternatives-to-infant-rice-cereal-a8571897937.

10. Jonathan Aviv, *The Acid Watcher Diet: A 28-Day Reflux Prevention and Healing Program* (New York: Harmony Books, 2017).

11. "Baby Foods Are Tainted with Dangerous Levels of Arsenic, Lead, Cadmium, and Mercury," *Staff Report: Subcommittee on Economic and Consumer Policy Committee on Oversight and Reform*, U.S. House of Representatives, February 4, 2021, https://oversight.house.gov/sites/democrats.oversight.house.gov/files/2021-02-04%20ECP%20Baby%20Food%20Staff%20Report.pdf.

12. Mac & Cheese with Chicken & Vegetables, Gerber, accessed on November 4, 2022, https://www.gerber.com/gerber-lil-meals-mac-cheese-with-chicken-for-toddlers.

13. American Academy of Pediatrics, "How to Reduce Added Sugar in Your Child's Diet: AAP Tips," Healthychildren.org, last modified April 2021, https://www.healthychildren.org/English/healthy-living/nutrition/Pages/How-to-Reduce-Added-Sugar-in-Your-Childs-Diet.aspx.

14. Natalie Jacewicz, "What Is 'Fruit Concentrate,' Anyway? And Is It Good for You?" NPR, last modified September 1, 2017, https://www.npr.org/sections/thesalt/2017/09/01/545336956/what-is-fruit-concentrate-anyway-and-is-it-good-for-you.

Chapter 2

1. Jessica Almy, J.D., M.S., and Margo G. Wootan, D.Sc., "Temptation at Checkout," Center for Science in the Public Interest, August 2015 https://www.cspinet.org/temptation-checkout.

2. "Acesulfame potassium," Center for Science in the Public Interest, accessed on November 4, 2022, https://www.cspinet.org/article/acesulfame-potassium.

3. "Sucralose," Center for Science in the Public Interest, accessed on November 4, 2022, https://www.cspinet.org/article/sucralose.

4. Monica Watrous, "Kellogg to Remove Artificial Colors, Flavors from Cereal," *Food Business News*, August 4, 2015, https://www.foodbusinessnews.net/articles/6576-kellogg-to-remove-artificial-colors-flavors-from-cereal.

5. Vani Hari, "I Infiltrated the Kellogg's Shareholders Meeting and What the CEO Said Will Shock You (VIDEO)," Food Babe, May , 2020, https://foodbabe.com/i-infiltrated-the-kelloggs-shareholders-meeting-and-what-the-ceo-said-will-shock-you-video.

6. Erin Hahn, et al., "Children Are Unsuspecting Meat Eaters: An Opportunity to Address Climate Change," *Journal of Environmental Psychology* 78 (December 2021), https://www.sciencedirect.com/science/article/pii/S0272494421001584.

7. "Glutamate," Cleveland Clinic, last reviewed April 25, 2022, https://my.clevelandclinic.org/health/articles/22839-glutamate.

8. Russell L. Blaylock, M.D., *Excitotoxins: The Taste That Kills*, (Health Press, 1994).

9. Carlos Ea Chagas, Marcelo M. Rogero, and Lígia A. Martini, "Evaluating the Links Between Intake of Milk/Dairy Products and Cancer," *Nutrition Reviews*, 70(5):294–300, May 1, 2012, https://doi.org/10.1111/j.1753-4887 .2012.00464.x.

10. Mbarga Manga Joseph Arsène, et al., "The Public Health Issue of Antibiotic Residues in Food and Feed: Causes, Consequences, and Potential Solutions," *Vet World*, 15 no. 3 (March 2022): 662–671, https://pubmed .ncbi.nlm.nih.gov/35497952.

11. Tosin Thompson, "The Staggering Death Toll of Drug-Resistant Bacteria," *Nature*, January 31, 2022, https:// www.nature.com/articles/d41586-022-00228-x.

12. Stephen Perrine and Heather Hurlock, "Fat Epidemic Linked to Chemicals Run Amok," *NBC News*, March 8, 2010, https://www.nbcnews.com/health/health-news/fat-epidemic-linked-chemicals-run-amok-flna1c9443537.

13. Anna Novoselov, "These Pesticides May Increase Cancer Risk in Children," UCLA Fielding School of Public Health, September 13, 2022, https://ph.ucla.edu/news/press-release/2022/sep/these-pesticides-may -increase-cancer-risk-children.

14. "IARC Monograph on Glyphosate," International Agency for Research on Cancer, World Health Organization, https://www.iarc.who.int/featured-news/media-centre-iarc-news-glyphosate/.

15. Aristo Vojdani and Charlene Vojdani, "Immune Reactivity to Food Coloring," *Alternative Therapies in Health and Medicine* 21 (March 2015) Suppl 1: 52–62, https://pubmed.ncbi.nlm.nih.gov/25599186.

16. Laurel Curran, "EU Places Warning Labels on Foods Containing Dyes," *Food Safety News*, July 21, 2010, https://www.foodsafetynews.com/2010/07/eu-places-warning-labels-on-foods-containing-dyes/.

17. Andria Kades, "Titanium Dioxide Ban Comes into Force, Companies Have Six Months to Adjust", *Food Ingredients First*, January 10, 2022, https://www.foodingredientsfirst.com/news/titanium-dioxide-ban-comes -into-force-companies-have-six-months-to-adjust.html.

18. Erica Buoso, et al., "Endocrine-Disrupting Chemicals' (EDCs) Effects on Tumour Microenvironment and Cancer Progression: Emerging Contribution of RACK1," *International Journal of Molecular Sciences* 21 no. 23 (December 3, 2020), https://pubmed.ncbi.nlm.nih.gov/33287384.

19. Lifespan, "Nitrates May Be Environmental Trigger for Alzheimer's, Diabetes and Parkinson's Disease." *ScienceDaily*, July 6, 2009, www.sciencedaily.com/releases/2009/07/090705215239.htm.

20. Eloi Chazelas, et al., "Nitrites and Nitrates from Food Additives and Natural Sources and Cancer Risk: Results from the Nutrinet-Santé Cohort," *International Journal of Epidemiology* 51, no.4 (August 10, 2022): 1106– 1119, https://pubmed.ncbi.nlm.nih.gov/35303088.

21. "Butylated Hydroxyanisole CAS No. 25013-16-5," *Report on Carcinogens, Fifteenth Edition*, Department of Health and Human Services National Toxicology Program, December 21, 2021, https://ntp.niehs.nih.gov/ntp /roc/content/profiles//butylatedhydroxyanisole.pdf.

22. Iliana E. Sweis and Bryan C. Cressey, "Potential Role of the Common Food Additive Manufactured Citric Acid in Eliciting Significant Inflammatory Reactions Contributing to Serious Disease States: A Series of Four Case Reports," *Toxicol Reports* 5 (August 9, 2018): 808–812, https://pubmed.ncbi.nlm.nih.gov/30128297.

23. David Andrews, "Natural vs. Artificial Flavors: Synthetic Ingredients in Natural Flavors and Natural Flavors in Artificial flavors," Environmental Working Group, https://www.ewg.org/foodscores/content/natural-vs-artificial-flavors/.

24. "Healthy Kids 'Sweet Enough' without Added Sugars," The Nutrition Source, Harvard T. H. Chan School of Public Health, last modified August 23, 2016, https://www.hsph.harvard.edu/nutritionsource/2016/08/23/aha-added-sugar-limits-children.

25. Aristo Vojdani and Charlene Vojdani, "Immune Reactivity to Food Coloring," *Alternative Therapies in Health and Medicine* 21 (March 2015) Suppl 1: 52–62, https://pubmed.ncbi.nlm.nih.gov/25599186.

26. "American Academy of Pediatrics Says Some Common Food Additives May Pose Health Risks to Children," Healthychildren.org, last modified July 23, 2018, https://www.healthychildren.org/English/news/Pages/AAP-Says-Some-Common-Food-Additives-May-Pose-Health-Risks-to-Children.aspx.

27. "Food Additives," CBC News Food Safety FAQs, last modified September 29, 2008, https://www.cbc.ca/news2/background/foodsafety/additives.html.

28. "European Union: Titanium Dioxide Banned as a Food Additive in the EU," U.S. Department of Agriculture, USDA Foreign Agricultural Service, last modified March 3, 2022, https://www.fas.usda.gov/data/european-union-titanium-dioxide-banned-food-additive-eu.

29. Laurel Curran, "EU Places Warning Labels on Foods Containing Dyes," *Food Safety News*, last modified July 21, 2010, https://www.foodsafetynews.com/2010/07/eu-places-warning-labels-on-foods-containing-dyes.

30. Sarah Kobylewski and Michael Jacobson, "Food Dyes: A Rainbow of Risks," Center for Science in the Public Interest, June 2010, https://www.cspinet.org/sites/default/files/media/documents/resource/food-dyes-rainbow-of-risks.pdf.

31. Patrick Sauer, "How Goldfish Crackers Took Over the World." *Fast Company*, last modified December 19, 2018, https://www.fastcompany.com/90283202/how-goldfish-crackers-took-over-the-world.

32. Allison Johnson, "Drugs in Your Milk? Maybe, Unless It's Organic," Natural Resources Defense Council, last modified July 9, 2019, https://www.nrdc.org/experts/allison-johnson/drugs-your-milk-maybe-unless-its-organic.

33. David Murphy and Henry Rowlands, "Glyphosate: Unsafe on Any Plate," The Detox Project, accessed on November 4, 2022, https://detoxproject.org/wp-content/uploads/2022/08/Final-Report.pdf.

Chapter 3

1. Anahad O'Connor, "How to Break Out of the Children's Menu Trap: A New Book on Children's Food Offers Suggestions on How to Encourage Healthful Eating," *The New York Times*, last modified February 20, 2020, https://www.nytimes.com/2019/10/23/well/eat/Children-food-health.html.

2. Rishi Sriram, "Why Ages 2–7 Matter So Much for Brain Development," *Edutopia*, last modified June 24, 2020, https://www.edutopia.org/article/why-ages-2-7-matter-so-much-brain-development.

3. Jill Anderson, "The Benefit of Family Mealtime," *Harvard EdCast*, Harvard Graduate School of Education, last modified April 1, 2020. https://www.gse.harvard.edu/news/20/04/harvard-edcast-benefit-family-mealtime.

4. Xanna Burg, et al., "Effects of Longer Seated Lunch Time on Food Consumption and Waste in Elementary and Middle School–age Children: A Randomized Clinical Trial," *JAMA Network Open* (June 2021), https://jamanetwork.com/journals/jamanetworkopen/fullarticle/2781214.

Chapter 4

1. Red Apple Dining, "Breakfast and Lunch Ingredients List: Elementary Schools," Seminole County Public Schools, accessed November 4, 2022, http://fs3.scps.k12.fl.us/Nutrition/Ingredient%20List%20Elementary%20-%20Breakfast-Lunch.pdf.

2. Carolyn Heneghan, "Candy Crush: NCA Survey Says Halloween Candy Sales to Hit $2.6B." Food Dive, last modified October 7, 2015, https://www.fooddive.com/news/candy-crush-nca-survey-says-halloween-candy-sales-to-hit-26b/406886.

3. "Genetically Engineered Sugar Is a Trick, Not a Treat," Center for Food Safety, last modified October 31, 2015, https://www.centerforfoodsafety.org/blog/4110/genetically-engineered-sugar-is-a-trick-not-a-treat.

INDEX

NOTE: Page references in *italics* refer to photos of recipes.

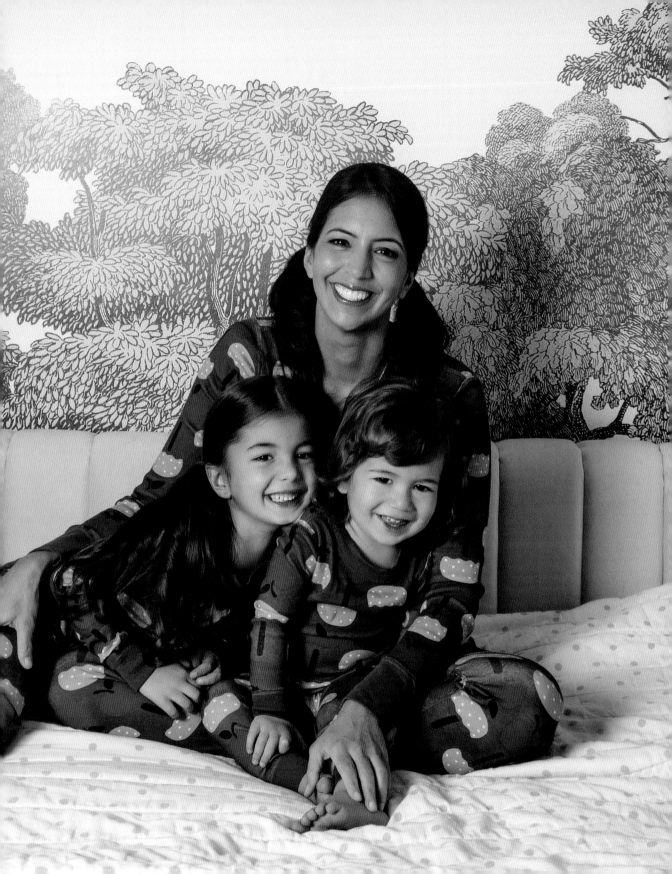

ACKNOWLEDGMENTS

To my amazing husband Finley. Your green thumb and ability to grow just about anything in our yard has been such a blessing to me and our children. Thank you for nurturing and taking care of the gorgeous golden berry plant on the cover of this book. Your brilliance in the garden I know has made our kids appreciate where food comes from.

To my children, your knowledge of the food industry will move mountains in your own health and all of those that you inspire with your way of eating. Our next generation will thank you.

To my dear son Bru, you are such a joy to be around. Your smile lights up my whole body. Thank you for being the challenge I needed to create solutions for tricky eating—especially while traveling.

To my daughter Harley, seeing you start to make your own dishes in our kitchen warms my heart. I love how open you are about trying new foods and your adventurous eating style. Taking you out to eat is one of my favorite things—we have so much fun!

To my mother, Veena. You show your love through cooking, and I see that I am inheriting that same trait as I am raising my children. Thank you for all the weekly drop offs of yummy homemade Indian meals.

To my dad, I am so thankful you are feeling vibrant and well with all of mom's daily cooking. You inspire me to keep writing books like this one.

To my father-in-law, Finley. Thank you for the never-ending jokes and laughter, you are truly one of a kind.

To my late mother-in-law, Diane. At the time, I never understood how much time and preparation you went through for our trips to the beach and mountains, but now, having my own children, I am forever grateful for all your tireless work. I will never forget all of the meals you made in advance of every trip to make sure we were all fed and didn't end up eating junk food. I miss you so much.

To Laura for always willing to get busy in the kitchen with me, your dedication to meal planning is an inspiration.

To my brother Yog, Judy, Summers, and Taylor. I love seeing the positive changes you've made in your lifestyles and your love of all the Truvani products.

To my Truvani team, for supporting the mission of creating real food snacks, products without toxins, and labels without lies.

To Sushila Melvani and Sri Aurobindo Society for the prayers and blessings.

To my amazing Food Babe Team - Kim and Pam. Your dedication and hardwork is inspiring millions, I am so lucky to have you both as co-workers. Kim you have a one-of-kind recipe styling eye that made each one of these pages come to life. Pam, your tireless questioning, edits and thoughtfulness that went into the making of this book is so appreciated.

To Susan Stripling, I will never get tired of working with you. You are a genius behind the camera and a true gem.

To Lisa, thanks for helping us all keep our smiles on during the photoshoots, I don't think I could have gotten through all of the family shots without you!

To my agents, Steve Troha and Scott Hoffman. Thank you for always being there for impromptu chats and for supporting me through the years.

To Reid Tracy, Patty Gift, and everyone at Hay House. I love being published by you. Thank you Sally Mason-Swaab for your beautiful insights that made this book complete.

To my recipe tester Sarah Tegnalia for your honest feedback and thoughtful modifications.

To all the mothers, fathers, and caregivers who strive to feed children daily. Your role is so important, I hope this book helps you, I wrote it for you.

ABOUT
THE AUTHOR

Named as one of the Most Influential People on the Internet by *Time Magazine*, **Vani Hari** is the revolutionary food activist behind foodbabe.com, co-founder of organic food brand Truvani, *New York Times* best selling author of *Food Babe Kitchen, The Food Babe Way*, and *Feeding You Lie*s. For most of her life, Vani ate whatever she wanted - candy, soda, fast food, processed food - until her typical American diet landed her where that diet typically does, in a hospital. Despite her successful career in corporate consulting, Hari decided that health had to become a priority. Her newfound goal drove her to investigate what is really in our food, how it is grown and what chemicals are used in its production. The more she learned, the more she changed and the better she felt.

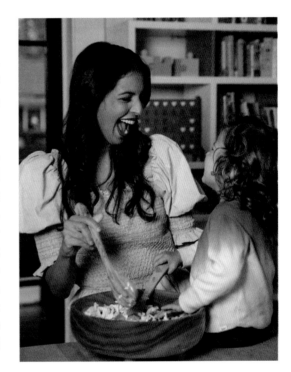

Encouraged by her friends and family, Hari started a blog called foodbabe.com in 2011. It quickly became a massive vehicle for change. She has led campaigns against food giants like Kraft, Starbucks, Chick-fil-A, Subway and General Mills that attracted more than 500,000 signatures and led to the removal of several controversial ingredients used by these companies. Through corporate activism, petitions, and social media campaigns, Hari and her Food Babe Army have become one of the most powerful populist forces in the health and food industries. Her drive to change the food system inspired the creation of her new company called Truvani, where she produces real food without added chemicals, products without toxins, and labels without lies. Hari has been profiled in the *New York Times* and *The Atlantic*, and has appeared on *Good Morning America*, *CBS This Morning*, *CNN*, *The Dr. Oz Show*, *The Doctors*, and *NPR*. Vani lives in Charlotte, North Carolina with her husband Finley and two children. Visit her online at: **foodbabe.com**

HAY HOUSE TITLES OF RELATED INTEREST

YOU CAN HEAL YOUR LIFE, the movie,
starring Louise Hay & Friends
(available as an online streaming video)
www.hayhouse.com/louise-movie

THE SHIFT, the movie,
starring Dr. Wayne W. Dyer
(available as an online streaming video)
www.hayhouse.com/the-shift-movie

* * *

*CRAZY SEXY KITCHEN: 150 Plant-Empowered Recipes to
Ignite a Mouthwatering Revolution*, by Kris Carr

*FOOD BABE KITCHEN: More Than 100 Delicious, Real Food
Recipes to Change Your Body and Your Life*, by Vani Hari

*MAKE YOUR OWN RULES COOKBOOK: More Than 100 Simple, Healthy Recipes
Inspired by Family and Friends Around the World*, by Tara Stiles

*THE SUGAR BRAIN FIX: The 28-Day Plan to Quit Craving the Foods T
hat Are Shrinking Your Brain and Expanding Your Waistline*, by Dr. Mike Dow

All of the above are available at your local bookstore,
or may be ordered by contacting Hay House (see next page).

* * *

We hope you enjoyed this Hay House book. If you'd like to receive our online catalog featuring additional information on Hay House books and products, or if you'd like to find out more about the Hay Foundation, please contact:

Hay House LLC, P.O. Box 5100, Carlsbad, CA 92018-5100
(760) 431-7695 or (800) 654-5126
www.hayhouse.com® • www.hayfoundation.org

———

Published in Australia by:
Hay House Australia Publishing Pty Ltd
18/36 Ralph St., Alexandria NSW 2015
Phone: +61 (02) 9669 4299
www.hayhouse.com.au

Published in the United Kingdom by:
Hay House UK Ltd
1st Floor, Crawford Corner,
91–93 Baker Street, London W1U 6QQ
Phone: +44 (0)20 3927 7290
www.hayhouse.co.uk

Published in India by:
Hay House Publishers (India) Pvt Ltd
Muskaan Complex, Plot No. 3,
B-2, Vasant Kunj, New Delhi 110 070
Phone: +91 11 41761620
www.hayhouse.co.in

———

Let Your Soul Grow

Experience life-changing transformation—one video
at a time—with guidance from the world's leading experts.

www.healyourlifeplus.com

NOTES

NOTES

NOTES

NOTES

NOTES

NOTES

NOTES

NOTES

NOTES